EAT LIKE A
HUMAN

EAT LIKE A HUMAN

NOURISHING FOODS AND ANCIENT WAYS OF COOKING TO REVOLUTIONIZE YOUR HEALTH

DR. BILL SCHINDLER

Little, Brown Spark
New York Boston London

It is unfortunate that we live in a world in which we need disclaimers for sharing information on how to nourish one another to achieve optimal health simply because it goes against the status quo — a status quo that is making us sicker every day. However, I have been advised that I need one here, and I would much rather present you with the information along with a disclaimer than not present the information at all.

The information in this book concerning selection and preparation of various foods is the product of my years of research and is provided for your information only. You should consult with appropriate health professionals on any matter relating to your health and well-being, including how you may react to any particular recipe or ingredient. —Bill Schindler

Little, Brown Spark
Hachette Book Group
1290 Avenue of the Americas, New York, NY 10104
littlebrownspark.com

First Edition: November 2021

Little, Brown Spark is an imprint of Little, Brown and Company, a division of Hachette Book Group, Inc. The Little, Brown Spark name and logo are trademarks of Hachette Book Group, Inc.

The publisher is not responsible for websites (or their content) that are not owned by the publisher.

The Hachette Speakers Bureau provides a wide range of authors for speaking events. To find out more, go to hachettespeakersbureau.com or call (866) 376-6591.

Photographs by Brianna Schindler
Illustrations by Sarah Schlick

ISBN 9780316244886
LCCN 20211936260

LSC-C

Printing 1, 2021

To my family: Christina, Brianna, Billy, and Alyssa.
I learned all of this for you. Thank you for inspiring me.

CONTENTS

EAT LIKE A
HUMAN

INTRODUCTION

Deep in central Kenya, amidst barren grasslands and bushwillows, days and miles from anything approaching modern "civilization," my family and I were about to drink blood. We were among the Samburu, semi-nomadic warrior people of East Africa who herd cattle, goats, and other livestock, and whose diets depend on a combination of raw milk and fresh blood drawn daily from the teats and necks of their animals.

After days of travel, we had come to a remote river village to witness and share in this practice. The final leg of our journey was driving for an hour up the middle of a wadi, or dried riverbed, since anything resembling a road had disappeared long ago. We arrived in the late afternoon, and the land shimmered with heat. Only the hum of insects broke the quiet.

Three young Samburu warriors stood sentry over the entrance to the trail that led to their village. They all wore brightly colored traditional attire, and their physiques were striking. In fact, for all of my travels around the world I had never encountered anyone who looked as healthy. Tall, lean, and muscular, they had broad faces split with wide smiles of straight, gleaming teeth. Their eyes were white and their skin glowed. And they looked this way despite a diet of very little meat, fruits, or vegetables. They had no access to supplemental vitamins, grocery stores, health care, nutritionists, or even fluoride. How did they do it? What was their secret? As an experimental archaeologist and food anthropologist, I wanted to find out.

I had brought my family with me: my wife, Christina; 12-year-old son, Billy; and 10- and 14-year-old daughters, Alyssa and Brianna. We were ready, or we thought we were. Billy and the girls stood by nervously, at once spellbound and alarmed by what was about to transpire. We watched one of the tribesmen lead a cow forward. Another held its head, steadying it. The animal huffed, shuffling its hooves in the dust, and then stilled. It regarded us with dark, wet eyes.

Then everything happened quickly. With a practiced dart of the wrist and a small bow and arrow crafted just for this purpose, one man efficiently pierced the cow's jugular. A second caught the blood flowing from the cow's neck in a gourd, about a liter. A third patched the small wound with dirt. Then the creature was released. It ambled off into the brush, unperturbed and seemingly unaffected. The tiny wound was not meant to kill the cow but rather to release a relatively small amount of blood, similar to the way we humans donate at a blood bank. The Samburu view blood the way most of the world views milk—as a renewable resource of high-quality nutrition.

In the moments that followed, one of the men filled a second gourd with fresh milk and then poured the two fluids, milk and blood, back and forth from one gourd to the other, mixing them thoroughly.

Finally, he handed the gourd to me. The moment had come.

I paused, looking out across the boundless savanna, the land stretching past the river, over expanses of whistling thorn and star grass. Then I looked down at the gourd, lifted it up, and took my first swallow of fresh blood.

What surprised me was how good it felt in my mouth—its density, warmth, and even flavor, akin to a rich chocolate milkshake with a little iron and salt thrown in. And after a few more swallows, it felt satiating. With very little, my body felt full and satisfied, almost as if it instinctively knew that it had just received a huge dose of nutrients that it could really do something with.

I passed the gourd to Christina, who swallowed and widened her eyes, feeling the same. Billy, who is always ready to jump in with both feet, took a healthy swig, but Brianna's was tiny, a mere taste. "Take a real sip," I encouraged her gently, and she did. But my youngest, Alyssa, couldn't be persuaded. She'd been afraid the cow was going to be hurt (or worse), and it was too far a cultural divide and too big a personal step for her to take.

This was OK, too. As the dusk gathered, we stood together in amazement of this place and these people, talking about what we had shared.

So why, you might ask, would I bring my family to this remote African bush to drink blood and milk with a group of Samburu warriors? The answer is both complicated and simple. Today, our relationship to food is filled with confusion and insecurity. Vegan or carnivore? Vegetarian or gluten-free? Keto or Mediterranean? Fasting or Paleo? Every day we hear about a new ingredient or food that is good or bad, a new diet that promises us everything. Our conversations are filled with a dizzying array of perspectives on our relationship to this most essential element of being human: food.

What if I told you that none of these dietary labels mattered? That you should never exclude a food source, no matter how alien or strange? What if I told you that you do not need to count calories, measure your portions, go hungry, or feel deprived? And, at the same time, that you can eat in such a way that you can become healthier, lose the extra pounds, live a more pain-free and energetic life, and contribute to the health of our planet?

How? By learning to eat like a human again. Simply put, this means finding food that is as nutrient-dense as possible, and preparing that food using methods that render it safe and make its nutrients available to our bodies. That's it. Whatever diet you follow, whatever your food preferences, the goal is to find and prepare food so that it provides the most nutrients. Eating in this way will maximize your health and simultaneously simplify the process of knowing how, what, and when to eat.

Our ancestors knew how to do this. Millions of years ago, they figured out how to eat in highly nutritious ways that allowed them to thrive. Today, our modern food systems have evolved away from this instinctive approach to food, even though we continue to inhabit bodies with the same needs as our ancestors'. This has been much to our detriment as a species.

Fortunately, there are still people in pockets of the world who continue to eat like humans. They employ ancient and traditional technologies to produce food of astounding nutrition, using everything from fermentation to cooking in mineral-rich dirt. For years I studied these kinds of foods and methods of preparation and taught them at Washington College in Chestertown, Maryland, where I created the Eastern Shore Food Lab, an innovative teaching, learning, and production space. I traveled the world, sometimes with my family, from the Mongolian steppes to the Kenyan savanna to the jungles of Thailand, to learn in person from the people who actually practice what I had studied, and to nourish myself using the same foods, tools, and methods as our ancestors. As I did so, I began to feel strong, healthy, and wildly alive, and it confirmed for me that this is the foundation of a healthy human diet. It made real all the work I had been doing for decades. My family and I adopted some of these foods and methods of preparation, and we all benefited from improved health.

As this book will lay out, today we can all be modern hunter-gatherers who use the same fundamental strategies our ancestors did to make their food safe, nutritious, and bioavailable, rather than succumbing to today's socially and economically driven norms. Our parents and grandparents were familiar with some of these foods, such as liver or sauerkraut; but others challenge our modern beliefs about what is food. You may not want to go as far as I have gone — drinking cow's blood mixed with raw milk, for instance — but in this book I will ask you to consider pushing your concepts and boundaries of what constitutes food, and I'll provide valid reasons for doing so. I will also provide some alternatives for those who aren't ready to stretch their boundaries as far. That said, as unusual or even off-putting as these foods might seem to most of us, they have enormous health benefits. For example, think about this: 100 grams of cricket flour contains 65 grams of protein, compared to just 32 grams of protein in the same amount of beef. Cricket flour includes all nine essential amino acids, has more calcium than milk, and has more iron than spinach. (A side benefit is that insects emit fewer greenhouse gases than most livestock, they can be raised almost anywhere, and production doesn't require massive water resources or large tracts of land, let alone clearing of land.)

An understanding of cultural context is key to this approach.

Even though we, as humans, have been biologically the same for some 300,000 years, we are culturally entirely different. This may seem obvious, but in the context of applying ancestral and traditional technologies and processes to food, it's an important point. For years, I didn't get this, and subjected my family to conflict and frustration as I insisted on certain rules that didn't take cultural context into consideration. This insistence began to manifest in me as a form of orthorexia — an obsession with eating only foods that one believes are healthy — and I created categories of "good foods" versus "bad foods" that provoked anxieties about food for everyone in my family. (In Chapter 9, "Sugar," I'll elaborate on these issues and how I came to grips with them.)

Eventually, after years of being obsessive in the extreme — refusing to eat birthday cake at a friend's celebration, demanding that my parents not give our kids any candy or sugary treats — I began to see the flaws in this approach and what it had to teach me about cultural context and compromise. We, as a family, found solutions — even sugary ones, which I explore in detail in Chapter 9 — that allowed for cultural acceptance without sacrificing the best-quality and most-nutritious foods. It's important to remember that food is more than nutrition. It is also a cultural experience that is invaluable to our health and happiness.

Chapter 1 describes our physical and cultural evolution through time as it relates to food. The chapters that follow discuss different food groups, like plants, animals, and dairy; explain preparation and cooking techniques associated with them; and provide concrete takeaways, recipes, and ideas on how to incorporate this information into modern life. The recipes range from easy (suitable for beginners) to advanced (for the more adventuresome). In each case, I will demonstrate the inseparable relationship between ancient and traditional technologies and today's food and health.

A word about terminology: The term *technology* as used in this book is not limited by our modern conception of the word. Instead, I use it to describe tools and processes that allow us to overcome our physical limitations to safely access food and its nutrients. For our forebears, primitive tools such as the sharp edge of a stone tool, a fire, or even a digging stick were technologies that they developed to help them access and prepare food. For us, it could mean the food processor in your cupboard or the blender on your countertop. The acts of fermenting, cooking, hunting, or even using a substance such as dirt in our food preparation fall into this definition as well. Likewise, the concept of processing food in this book has nothing to do with "processed foods" as we know them today.

I realize that overhauling our diets and changing our relationship with food is not going to happen overnight, and some of us may never get over our aversion to certain unfamiliar foods or have the time to use all of the methods I describe. I get that. I'm not suggesting that we all start drinking cow's blood milkshakes daily. What I do hope, however, is to offer you basic steps that incrementally build on one another to reconnect you with your food and increase the safety and nourishment of your diet. Whether this means inspiring you to start eating or cooking in new ways, or to simply start thinking about food differently as you stroll the grocery store aisles, it is all transformative and ultimately empowering in our common goal of seeking good health — and a healthy planet.

Chapter 1

ASKING THE RIGHT QUESTIONS:

NOT JUST WHAT, BUT HOW?

It was the opportunity of a lifetime. I was starring in National Geographic's *The Great Human Race,* a television series in which I was tasked with finding food and shelter using only the tools available during particular time periods of our evolution as humans. In Tanzania, I replicated a 2.5-million-year-old Oldowan tool kit to scavenge meat from a carcass on the savanna as fast as I could, before the lions returned. In Mongolia, I used bone and stone tools to hunt rabbit; and in the Republic of Georgia, I replicated a 40,000-year-old spear point to take down a wild boar with an atlatl. I felt hunger, I felt fear, I felt fierce joy and relief when I successfully hunted or found wild food that sustained me.

But now, here I was in Alaska, ostensibly in a bitter winter some 15,000 years ago, when our ancestors were attempting to cross what was then the Bering Land Bridge from Asia to North America. After two days of barely surviving with no food on the Arctic tundra, where ripping winds drove snow across endless miles of ice-glittered scrub, my co-star and I had walked south far enough for the snow to change to an icy rain, and before us was a pond with a beaver lodge. We desperately needed protein and fat to keep going, and I scouted the pond edge to find a place to set a primitive snare to trap a beaver. Once I found it, I knew my choices were stark: go into the freezing pond buck naked and then put my dry clothing back on; go into the pond fully clothed and come out in sopping deerskin clothes, risking hypothermia at best, death at worst; or, finally, not go into the pond at all and spend another night sleepless and starving.

God, I was cold! My hands were freezing up as I frantically worked to prepare as much of the trap as I could before stripping down and wading in to set the critical anchor — three atlatl darts I would stab into the bottom of the pond to form a kind of tripod, and to which I would attach the snare's anchor line. Behind me the mountains loomed like gray giants of mist, fog, and rock, the sky a leaden menace threatening more snow any minute.

You might think that at this point, all I was worried about was success-fully setting the trap and getting my freezing butt out of the water and back to a warm fire. You'd be wrong. What was freaking me out was not the cold, the hunger, or even the way my steaming breath was coming in gasps and my limbs shook uncontrollably. It was the fact that I was about to get naked in front of an entire production crew, two cameras, and a drone. Let's be honest: This was a television show. If I failed to find food, the crew wasn't going to let me die out here. But my commitment to this project was to take it as close to the edge as possible — to truly begin to grasp the challenges that our ancestors faced and overcame — and that meant strip-ping and walking into a freezing pond in front of all these people (and knowing that this scene would be aired before millions of viewers). And I have never felt comfortable taking even my *shirt* off in public. Ever.

If you watch this episode, you'll see that I look strong, athletic, ripped. But it wasn't always this way — far from it. And the fear I was feeling at this moment drew deep from what had been, for so much of my life, my unhealthy relationship with food. It's a story I suspect many of you can relate to in some form or another. As a chubby, awkward kid, I was picked on for my size. I didn't feel like food was something that nourished me. Food was something that scared me. It was something that made me fat. It was something that made other kids make fun of me. Then I became a wrestler in high school, eventually making the varsity team at one of the country's top Division 1 college programs. And I traded one unhealthy relationship with food for another. Food became something that prevented me from making my competitive weight. I binged and purged and fought with food—repeatedly and regularly losing and regaining more than 20 pounds a week! And after college and wrestling, the weight piled on with a vengeance, and I became an overweight adult. With that came health issues like irritable bowel syndrome, metabolic syndrome, even joint pain. All the while, I was constantly—to the point of obsession—trying to figure out what to eat. Over decades of research that encompassed prehistoric and experimental archaeology and took me from fieldwork with indigenous and traditional peoples around the world to the professional kitchens of global Michelin star chefs, I sought to answer that question: "What should I eat?" And I began to find the answers only when I realized that, all along, *that's not the only question I should have been asking.*

While we all are asking *"What* should I eat?" the equally—if not more—important question that must accompany this is *"How* should I eat?" Most people will take the latter question quite literally, as in "What time should I eat?" or "How much should I eat?" or "Should I eat slowly?" But in the context of this book, I'm going to ask you to expand your thinking about this word beyond those literal questions. Instead, I'm going to ask you to consider *how* as a concept that is directly connected to what our ancestral dietary past can teach us about our relationship to food today. In the introduction, I asked you to think about the word *technology* in a much broader way than is typical, to include everything from the high-speed blender on your kitchen counter to a Paleolithic stone tool or fire. *"How* should I eat?" requires a similar rethinking. Focusing on *how* means reconnecting to specific processes and technologies that we apply to our food from the moment we acquire it to the moment we put it in our mouths. This is where we have the opportunity to make the most, nutritionally speaking, of our food—or not. Our modern human predicament is that today we can eat to obesity and still be malnourished. This reality has everything to do with the ways we as individuals, as well as our cultures and food systems, have strayed from that fundamental dietary imperative of our ancestors: *how* to eat the safest, most nutrient-dense, bioavailable foods possible. Hewing to that imperative is literally what made us human and is the focus of this book. To begin to understand it, we have to shift some perspectives and go back in time.

First, the perspective shift.

Figuring out how to eat is a challenge unique to humans. Think about it. No other animal asks this question. No other animal hires nutritionists or doctors to provide dietary advice. No other animal wastes its energy eating foods that provide zero nutritional or digestive value. And much of our ancestors' efforts to figure out how to eat were efforts to overcome what were — and still are — fundamental biological and physical weaknesses that we humans have always struggled to surmount. People don't like to hear this, but when viewed through the prism of this most basic need — food — we humans are one of the weakest species on the planet, and this simple, uncomfortable fact has direct bearing on how we must feed ourselves differently than every other animal.

But wait, you'll say. Look at athletes like Usain Bolt, Arnold Schwarzenegger, and Michael Phelps. There's nothing weak about physical specimens like these! Well, let's measure them next to some cousins from the animal kingdom. The Federation of American Societies for Experimental Biology reports that relative to body length, the fastest animal on earth is a southern Californian mite that can move at 322 times its body length per second. Researchers Robert J. Knell and Leigh W. Simmons discovered that a dung beetle can pull 1,141 times its own body weight, making it pound for pound the strongest animal on the planet. Fisheries biologist Dave Kerstetter recorded sailfish reaching speeds of up to 68 miles per hour, making these fish the fastest swimmers in the world. How do our human athletes stack up? To keep up with that southern Californian mite, Usain Bolt would have to run 1,300 miles per hour. To outlift that dung beetle, Arnold Schwarzenegger would have to pull six double-decker buses full of people. To pass that sailfish, Michael Phelps would have to cover 2,800 meters in the time it normally takes him to swim 200.

I use these examples simply to shift your thinking a little, because to begin to understand how we as humans must learn to eat, you first have to understand that our physical weakness compared to other species means we are far less capable of obtaining food from our environment. For our ancestors, this was a matter of life and death. They couldn't run as fast as other animals, they couldn't fly, they couldn't even dig into the ground as well as other species.

The second reality to understand is how biologically deficient we were, and are, as a species. Other animals are built to digest what they consume, and their diets match what they're biologically equipped to handle. Herbivores like cows, for instance, are custom-built to process tough vegetal material like grass with their multi-chambered digestive systems. In a specially designed chamber called the rumen, microbial fermentation begins to break down food that eventually returns to the cow's mouth, where mechanical processing resumes with cud-chewing. (Picture the placid, Zen nature of a cow chewing its cud and you can easily see where the word *ruminate*—which stems from the Latin *ruminor*, "chew over again"—found its contemporary meaning: to think deeply and slowly about something.) Ducks, geese, and other grain-eating birds are perfectly designed to safely digest seeds, thanks to their crop (a specialized expansion of their esophagus), where grains are temporarily stored to slowly ferment and break down. From there, the grains travel to the gizzard, where they're ground between two muscular disks.

But what about us? The harsh reality is that biologically speaking, we have no business eating almost any food that we consume (more on this in a minute). In fact, other than when we are infants and well equipped to drink mother's milk, the only foods our digestive tracts are biologically *designed* to consume are the insects and limited amounts of wild fruits and vegetables that made up the diets of our early ancestors. How we overcame these physical and biological deficiencies and learned how to eat is the story of how our ancestors became human both culturally and biologically. Simply put: We developed technologies to do outside of our bodies what other animals do naturally inside theirs. Through serendipity, imitation, innovation, or some combination thereof, we created tools and behavior patterns that allowed us to access foods from our environment that otherwise would have been unavailable to us—whether physically or biologically—and we learned how to make them as safe, nutrient-dense, and bioavailable as possible for our weak, inefficient bodies *before we ate them*. This quest for safe, nourishing foods drove everything we did.

So, how did we physically evolve, and how did our relationship with food and food technologies change during that evolution?

Five to seven million years ago, our ancestors were gatherers, subsisting primarily on diets of seasonally available wild fruits and vegetables, and probably some insects as a source of protein. This limited diet was enough to sustain their small bodies and brains. *Australopithecus afarensis* (better known as the fossilized bones discovered in 1974 and nicknamed "Lucy") lived from about 3.9 to 2.9 million years ago. This species was about 3.5 feet tall and weighed about 70 pounds, with a brain about the size of a fist. By 300,000 years ago, when *Homo sapiens*—that is, us—first appeared, on average we stood about 5 feet tall and weighed about 130 pounds. Perhaps most significantly, our brains had undergone a 360 percent increase in size from Lucy's.

So, over millions of years, our brains and bodies grew larger. But the story becomes more complicated when we look at other physical changes over time. Our teeth, for instance, were growing smaller. If you look at the jaw of *Homo habilis*—that's an ancestor from some 2.5 million years ago—you'll see huge molars, almost three times the size of the molars in our mouths today. Teeth are one of the few anatomical features we have that allow us to mechanically break down food—and they were *shrinking*. Likewise, our guts were also getting smaller. We know this by looking at the ribcage; in *Australopithecus afarensis,* the ribcage widens as it descends, making room for what was still a relatively modest-size gut. In *Homo sapiens,* on the other hand, the ribcage tapers as it reaches its base, indicating a smaller gut size. In fact, our digestive tracts today are a little more than half of what would be expected for similar-size primates. Why is this significant? Because a smaller gut means a less efficient digestive system. The size of our digestive tract is directly proportional to the amount of food we can consume and the amount, types, and quality of the nutrition that our body will absorb.

So, what was going on here? Even as our bodies and our brains—the most nutritionally expensive organ in our bodies—were growing, other physical attributes responsible for transforming the food we eat into nutrients that our bodies could use to fuel that growth were diminishing or, in some cases, disappearing entirely. How could that happen?

The beginning of the answer to that question dates to about 3.3 million years ago. I picture it occurring something like this:

Some of our ancestors, most likely *Australopithecus afarensis,* are crouched behind an acacia tree somewhere just west of what's now called Lake Turkana in Kenya. They are staring longingly at a fresh animal kill, having recently watched a saber-toothed cat take down this prey, rip it apart with canines designed specifically for the task, and gorge itself on the nutrient-rich blood, fat, and offal inside. Once satiated, the cat has done what predators often do in this situation — ambled off to take a nap and digest the feast. This is the moment when our ancestors can swoop in and try to steal some meat left behind before other scavengers take over or the lion returns for seconds. Until now, they could barely get any meaningful quantity of meat off the bones before the scavengers or predators returned. They were thwarted by their physical limitations — teeth too small and dull to effectively tear meat from a carcass, muscles too weak to pull apart limbs, fingernails too ineffectual to scrape anything more than a morsel. Determined and desperate, these particular ingenious ancestors use the one biological advantage they do possess, their brain. Perhaps one of them picks up two rocks, smashes them together, and in less than a second produces a durable, razor-sharp edge. Another does the same. Armed with the world's first knives, they rush in, hack off chunks of meat bigger than anything they've ever been able to scavenge before, and carry them back to their group to share.

This was a transformative moment in the history of our species. In that one simple act, our ancestors created the first tool, transcending their physical limitations and interacting with their environment and food in an entirely new and powerful way. This tool essentially mimicked what the teeth and claws of those majestic apex predators could accomplish as a matter of course. It marked the first time that we as humans started figuring out not just what to eat, but how to eat it. It put us on the trajectory that has led us from being the weakest species on the planet to the top of the food chain.

These tools introduced meat into our ancestors' diets (which means that we have been eating meat for almost 3.5 million years). And while it was unequivocally a major advance, since meat is certainly packed with far more nutrients than the fruits and vegetables that people at this time had access to, we were still scavenging. Though we had some access to bones and the vitally nutritious marrow within, by the time we got to a carcass even with our stone tools, the animal that had killed the prey had already devoured the most nutrient-dense parts—the organs, blood, and fat. Semantics makes a huge difference here. It was not the introduction of meat that made the biggest impact; rather, it was the introduction of *animals*. And the next great technological innovations that enabled our ancestors to gain first access to those animals—through hunting, fishing, and trapping—were critically important in our dietary evolution, because for the first time, we had first dibs on the most nutrient-dense parts of the animal. No longer were we scavenging leftover meat from a carcass. Now, as hunter-gatherers, we were predators ourselves, able to bring down our own prey and keep and use all of the animal.

The current earliest examples of hunting in the archaeological record— the fossilized remains of 2-million-year-old animal carcasses near Lake Victoria in Kenya, as well as remains in Olduvai Gorge in Tanzania—date to approximately 1.8 million years ago. By studying how modern predators like lions and cheetahs behave, archaeologists were able to determine that such carnivores hadn't killed these animals; rather, intentional human hunting had. The first direct evidence of hunting dates to approximately 400,000 years ago in Schöningen, Germany. In the mid-1990s, archaeologists discovered eight wooden spears buried with approximately 16,000 animal bones. Expertly crafted from conifers (all spruce except for one made from pine), these spears resemble modern javelins and, given some of the physical characteristics their crafters bestowed on them—including the intentional location of the center of gravity—they likely were designed to be thrown. Their direct association with so many animal bones, almost all of them belonging to an ancient form of horse, *Equus mosbachensis,* and many of them exhibiting butchering marks, indicates that they were used for hunting.

The introduction of hunting, fishing, and trapping transformed us biologically and culturally. Technological advancements such as spears, atlatls, slings, and bows allowed us to hunt from a relatively safe distance. Nets, traps, weirs, and poisons gave us the ability to capture large quantities of fish with relatively little effort. Deadfalls, snares, and pit traps did our work for us, letting us allocate our time to other important activities.

Many of the hunting technologies we developed overcame our biological limitations by mimicking something that other animals do naturally. We're slow and earthbound, but we developed complex weapon systems that let us cover a long distance almost instantly by accurately launching projectiles into the air. We don't have large canines, so we created stone tools to act as our teeth. But, at about the same time we started developing these new technologies to imitate how animals hunt and eat, we did something that no other animal has ever done: We created a way to cook our food.

If you really stop to think about it, the fact that we humans associate with fire at all is very strange indeed. Most animals are deathly afraid of fire and go out of their way to avoid it. Our ancestors' association with fire is a much more complicated story than simply learning how to harness its power and control it. The first thing we had to do was learn how not to be afraid of it. University of Toronto anthropologist Frances D. Burton, who wrote *Fire: The Spark That Ignited Human Evolution,* believes that it took millions of years to build a solid enough relationship with fire to even reach the point where we could learn to harness and control it. According to her, the process may have begun as early as six million years ago, when our brave and perhaps reckless pre-human ancestors first approached natural fires on the African savanna. This first and continued contact would have allowed them to comprehend the advantages of fire in offering food, protection, warmth, and light. Eventually, over millions of years, our ancestors began to understand how fire works and what happens to it when it runs out of fuel. Over time, perhaps they learned to nurture fire by providing it with grass or twigs. According to Burton's theory, this long process set the stage for our ability to control and create fire, at will, approximately two million years ago.

As you can imagine, the ephemeral nature of fires, especially small, single-use fires, makes them difficult to identify in the archaeological record, and the timing of fire's appearance in our past is a subject that remains controversial. However, evidence exists that lends support to the 2-million-year timeframe for this technological revolution. The current earliest evidence of intentional, human-created fire comes from a site in Koobi Fora, Kenya, where oxidized patches of earth, altered in color and texture in a way that's possible only through contact with heat in the presence of oxygen, date to between 1.6 and 1.8 million years ago. At the Chesowanja site in Kenya, archaeologists have recovered burned clay clasts, chemically and physically transformed by fire, that date to 1.4 million years ago. Two caves in South Africa provide even more solid evidence. At Swartkrans Cave, remains of burnt bones date to between 1 and 1.5 million years ago, while at Wonderwerk Cave, remains of ash and carbonized pieces of leaves, wood, and bone date to approximately 1 million years ago.

Proxy, or representative, evidence also corroborates this theory. Harvard University primatologist Richard Wrangham, who wrote *Catching Fire: How Cooking Made Us Human,* believes that *Homo erectus* would have required a diet that consisted at least in part of cooked food in order to support its large body despite its tooth size. Part of his research has shown that to subsist on a completely raw, unprocessed diet, we would have to have spent 42 percent of our day simply chewing. Cooking meat, for instance, allows us to obtain its nutrients with far less work and time. It's also interesting to note that the first migration out of Africa that began around 1.7 million years ago, one that witnessed *Homo erectus* traveling into northern latitudes, would have been possible only by relying on the heat of a fire to maintain safe body temperatures. The fact that this migration was occurring at the beginning of the Pleistocene, or the last ice age, further confirms the need for an external, and portable, source of heat and light.

Wrangham believes that the introduction of fire and cooking technology into the human diet was so powerful that it is actually the primary driver responsible for us becoming human as we know it. Cooking transformed our ancestral diets in extremely powerful ways and dramatically expanded the breadth of our diets. Through cooking, foods that harbor harmful bacteria or heat-sensitive toxins can be rendered safe to eat.

Cooking begins the breakdown of proteins and starches, making the nutrients found in meat and root-based foods like tubers and rhizomes easier for the human body to absorb — and, in some cases, providing the only way our bodies can have access to certain nutrients. Cooking concentrates nutrients, rendering them denser, and it makes food more enticing by altering color, flavor, and smell. Hunting and cooking were the most powerful influences on our ancestral diets that humans would see until the Agricultural Revolution. It's no coincidence that the monumental nutrient density and bioavailability that this dynamic duo introduced to the human diet occurred simultaneously with the most dramatic increases in brain, body, and population sizes that our genus *Homo* has ever experienced.

The technological revolution that began when our ancestors struck two rocks together to form a sharp-edged tool continued to expand and grow over the next two million years. Our ancestors became experts at developing ways to transform foods that had been biologically or physically unavailable to us. In addition to becoming hunters and gaining first access to the most nutrient-dense parts of animals, we learned how to detoxify and process plants outside our bodies. We developed advanced forms of cooking, fermentation, curing, and nixtamalization (an ancient way to process corn that we will discuss in depth in Chapter 5, "Maize") to benefit from more digestible nutrition. We invented strategies to pre-digest almost every food in the world, such as intentional fermentation of vegetables (sauerkraut), dairy (cheese, yogurt, and butter), and grains (sourdough bread and beer). We learned how to create storage vessels and technologies, including curing meats, that let us capitalize on surplus from a successful hunt or harvest; in fact, some of our storage techniques, like lacto-fermentation (used to produce foods such as yogurt and kimchi), enhanced food's nutrient density and bioavailability. These technological advances supported everything we attempted to do. Populations grew as we expanded across the globe and used our developing technologies to exploit new and diverse food resources to their fullest potential, no matter the environment or geography in which we found ourselves.

It's worth it to stop here and consider this simple truth that the archaeological record lays bare for us: Everything that our ancestors did in terms of food was geared toward efficiently obtaining it and learning how to process it so that our bodies could safely draw the most nutrition from it. Through fulfilling that clear imperative, we became more and more viscerally connected with our food—how to access it and, most important, how to prepare it for our bodies.

When we began to stray from this, we began slowly and surely to grow increasingly distanced from our food. This shift began as we became food producers about 15,000 years ago with the Agricultural Revolution, and it accelerated when we became food consumers—that is, when our emphasis shifted from growing to purchasing our food, beginning with the Industrial Revolution in the 1700s. With this growing distance, we began to lose our hard-earned food knowledge and, I would argue, we put ourselves on the exact opposite trajectory from our ancestors. Today, rather than growing in health and well-being, we are struggling with a multitude of illnesses and maladies directly related to poor diets, malnutrition, and misinformation. Few of us have any direct connection to producing our own food, or even to those who produce our food. Our culture and economies have shifted so dramatically over time that it is all too common for us to work all day to make money to go to a store to buy food grown, processed, and delivered by corporations and people we don't know. We haven't seen the farm, walked the crop rows, touched the animals, met the farmer, butcher, plant manager, or truck driver. More important, they haven't met us. In that anonymity, they bear little or no responsibility to us or to our health and welfare. And in our detachment from our foods' sources, we willingly hand over our own power and ability to more safely and sustainably control every aspect of the food we eat.

Meanwhile, cheap shortcuts in food preparation have permeated all aspects of our diet. Many of these small, incremental steps that have diminished the nutrient density, bioavailability, and, in some cases, safety of our food have made us sicker. In a twisted evolution of our 3.5-million-year-old quest for nutrient-dense foods, we now strive for nutrient-free foods. Think about it: Most packaged foods on American grocery store shelves boast about what they *don't* have in them—they're fat-free, gluten-free, dairy-free, lactose-free, calorie-free, carb-free. The message marketed to us is

"Go ahead, eat lots of food and don't feel bad because it won't make you fat or unhealthy." And so, we are obsessed with and confused by focusing on the single question: "What should I eat?"

When we include the critically important corollary — "How should I eat?" — we can more clearly understand that *what* we eat has to be considered along with *how* we approach it from the moment we acquire it to the moment we consume it.

By reconnecting to processes and technologies that let us maximize our food's nutritional value, we transform our concept of food. When we understand that how a food is processed is at least as important as what that food is, we can never again look at common categories of food such as bread, cheese, and meat in the same way. If, for example, you buy a popular brand of processed 100 percent whole wheat bread to feed your family, by our USDA food pyramid standards, you're making a good choice (and yes, it's far better than buying processed 100 percent enriched-flour white bread). But it is a poor nutritional choice compared to sourdough breads that rely on wild bacterial and yeast fermentations that leaven as well as detoxify and make nutrients more accessible to our bodies. By the same token, meat-based protein no longer means the pale whitish hunk of pre-seasoned pork tenderloin or chicken breast you find in your grocery store's meat case. Instead, it means that we should be eating all parts of an animal — meat, marrow, organs, even offal — to increase nutritional value and support the ethical, environmental, and economic advantages of a nose-to-tail strategy for eating animals. A package of American cheese or a container of yogurt may meet the standard for the dairy category of the food pyramid, but it bears zero resemblance, nutritionally or in terms of flavor and sustenance, to cheese or yogurt made with grass-fed (preferably raw) dairy and fermented using traditional methods to lower the amount of lactose while enhancing the probiotic load, vitamin content, and digestibility.

When we make our dietary decisions using this more holistic point of view, we eat foods that safely and sustainably nourish. When we eat them, we rise from the table feeling comforted, satiated, and fulfilled. We should not feel hungry, nor should we have to loosen our belts or reach for the antacid. This is how our ancestors ate, and this is what we should be striving for in our diets now. Of course, I'm not suggesting that we all learn how to hunt with an atlatl and butcher our catch with a hand-crafted obsidian blade (although trust me, it's fun and rewarding to try these technologies!). We may be essentially biologically the same — with the same nutritional needs — as we were 300,000 years ago, but we are living in the 21st century. Our expectations about how food should taste, smell, and look — and even the way we present it and gather to consume it — are entirely different. Our ability to incorporate ancestral and traditional food technologies into our busy, modern lives requires planning and time. Some of us have a lot more of the latter than others. Nor would I expect you, for instance, to trash everything in your pantry, dump out your refrigerator, and upend your life to make a radical change (in fact, I recommend against it). For some of you, even a small foray into the "how" of food may be sufficient. But if you're reading this book, I suspect that food and your relationship to it is a subject into which you've already put a lot of time and thought. And it's likely you have genuine concerns for how our diet impacts the world around us, perhaps even goals for sustainability, ethics, and economics in the way that we feed ourselves. For all of those reasons, I believe the diet of our future should absorb the lessons of our past and blend them with modern culinary arts and foodways to create a food system and philosophy that can meet our contemporary cultural expectations while creating foods that are deeply nourishing and sustainable.

On the Alaskan tundra, freezing in a beaver pond in a desperate attempt to find a calorie-rich, nutrient-dense meal, all of these realities were slamming into me — my childhood as a chubby kid burdened by a self-destructive relationship with food; my lifework of understanding primitive technologies and ancestral foodways so that I could better feed myself and my family; my yearning to know more about how our ancestors created the technologies to overcome so many physical deficiencies and beat the survival odds. The snare I was setting — using cordage I'd made from natural plant fibers and waterproofed with tallow — was a technology tens of thousands of years old. I stabbed a series of sticks into the mud near the bank to funnel the beaver toward the snare, whose loop was suspended in the water. My drenched hands and feet were already freezing, but after stripping off my deerskin clothes, it took me a bone-chilling five minutes or so waist-deep in the water to set the trap's anchors and properly adjust the snare. Once done, I flailed out of the water, still naked in front of all those cameras. I frantically reached for the clothes that I'd left hanging on a bush. My whole body was shaking, and as I stumbled back to the camp where my co-star, Cat, had been tending the fire that we'd built hours earlier with a bow-drill, my muscles were shutting down and my legs wobbled like Jell-O. But I knew, just as our ancestors did, that the trap would do its work as we stayed warm through the night by the fire.

The next morning, while I was still recovering from the chill, Cat walked to the pond, now brittle and glistening with a covering of ice. Beneath it, a beaver hung suspended, caught and drowned in the snare. Cat broke the ice and dragged the beaver to the pond's bank. Using a simple stone blade, she skinned and butchered the prize. Later, we cooked the fat-rich tail and nutrient-dense heart and organs over the fire. It was a deeply rejuvenating meal — physically, spiritually, and mentally. I realized that I was proud not only of successfully acquiring this unparalleled food source in a desperate situation, but of facing and overcoming that deep-seated discomfort in my body image driven by a destructive and misinformed relationship with food. What I was learning was how to begin asking the right questions, the ones we all are constantly compelled — through daily necessity and primitive, ancestral drive — to ask ourselves: not simply what should we eat, but how can we make our food as safe and nourishing as possible?

Chapter 2

PLANTS

SNACKS IN THE SIDEWALK

Plants should scare the hell out of you.

I realize this is counterintuitive to so much of what we're told about what we should eat. Most of us, when we walk through a grocery store's produce section, think: *This is where my health begins.* We believe we're on the right track when a spinach salad hits our plate at least a couple of times a week, when we choose the kale smoothie after our workout, when we steam extra servings of those stalks of suspiciously fresh-looking asparagus that show up in the grocery store just in time for Thanksgiving dinner. But it just isn't that easy, or that straightforward.

Whether in our grocery stores, our backyards, the hot heart of the Amazon basin, or the frigid barrens of the Arctic tundra, every plant on the planet contains toxins—among them phytates, tannins, cyanogenic glycosides, oxalates, saponins, lectins, and enzyme inhibitors. Some of them will kill you; some will just make you sick. Some won't hurt you at all, while others will build up—or "bioaccumulate"—in your body over time and cause issues later in life. Some of these toxins can be used as medicines, and some are actually good for you. But all plants have them. Spinach, for example, contains oxalates, which under a microscope and in your body resemble tiny shards of glass. We are only now beginning to understand that many ailments commonly diagnosed as inflammation, fibromyalgia, and even pseudogout (when calcium oxalate crystals build up in the joints and are mistaken for gout) can be attributed to plant toxins like oxalates. Sufferers of kidney stones, for instance, are warned to stay away from oxalates, because they can cause more stones.

Toxins in plants are designed to protect the plant; they are nature's pesticides, herbicides, and fungicides. And while we know that human-applied pesticides can be dangerous, it's eye-opening to note that pesticides produced by plants themselves actually account for 99.9 percent of pesticides that we eat. It's estimated that every American eats 1.5 grams of naturally occurring pesticides per day, which is about 10,000 times more than the amount of synthetic pesticides we eat. In other words, the plants themselves deliver more pesticides to our systems than what we spray on them. Through selective breeding and genetic modification, we have reduced naturally occurring toxins in today's produce, but we haven't extinguished them. And when we eat the same vegetables year-round, rather than only when they are in season—for instance, when we eat asparagus, a spring crop, at Thanksgiving—even these very small amounts of toxins can build up in our bodies and do us harm.

Manioc, also known as cassava or yucca and a staple for 700 million people worldwide, contains extremely toxic cyanogenic glycosides—a form of cyanide. The root, which also possesses high nutritional and medicinal qualities, requires extensive processing to be made safe to eat. It has been genetically modified to produce what's called sweet manioc, which has much lower levels of toxins (but also less nutrition). This is what you find in American grocery stores, but indigenous people of the Amazon basin still grow and subsist on the wild, toxic variety, using different methods of processing to make it safe. This allows for a more nutritious food that also has a nearly 100 percent crop yield because of its natural defenses.

I'm not saying we shouldn't eat plants. But throughout this book I'm asking you to rethink what you believe and have been told as it relates to our food and how we eat it. Your relationship with plants as food may be one of the most challenging to turn on its head. What have we all been told since we were kids? "Eat your vegetables!" Vegetables have been sold to us as the cornerstone of a lean, healthy diet, and they certainly confer health benefits. But they aren't nearly as good for you as our contemporary food system would have you believe. Plants were not put on the planet to feed us, nor are we biologically built to eat a vast majority of them. They are loaded with toxins and they don't easily give up their nutrition to our bodies. So, if we are going to eat plants, we need to ask the right question: *How do I make this plant as safe, nutritious, and accessible as I can?*

There are a few ways to answer this question. One is through the practice of foraging — which encompasses identifying a wild plant (which itself requires an understanding of seasonality), harvesting it properly, and safely preparing it to eat — and seeing how it can help us reevaluate and renew our relationship with plants. Sourcing vegetables directly, such as growing them yourself or purchasing them from a local farmer's market, is a positive step toward paying more attention to plant safety by connecting directly with a grower and choosing and eating only what's in season. But foraging takes this awareness to an entirely new, powerful level. Another strategy involves the suite of technologies we can use to make the nutrients in plants safe and available to our bodies through detoxification and processing. There are many, including nixtamalization (which we'll talk more about in Chapter 5), geophagy (we'll discuss this and potatoes in depth in Chapter 8), dehydrating, grinding, grating, and cooking. But we'll focus in this chapter on the game-changing technology of fermentation, an excellent example of an ancient processing skill that is easy to do in your modern kitchen. Both strategies — foraging and fermentation — accomplish the all-important goal of reconnecting us to our food, its sources, its preparation, and its value to us both nutritionally and culturally.

To start rethinking our relationship with plants as food, it helps to think like a plant. Like every other organism, plants are engaged in a constant fight to survive. Wild plants are wild because they have not been domesticated, meaning they haven't been genetically modified to adapt to a culturally created environment. Instead, these wild plants have evolved over eons to survive and thrive on their own so that they can fulfill the evolutionary imperative of all living things: to procreate and, by doing so, produce viable offspring that can do the same. To accomplish this, plants have developed complicated physical and chemical mechanisms to interact with the outside world. Among these are allelochemicals—chemical compounds created and released by the plant—which can be used for a variety of purposes. They can repel all sorts of bad actors, whether predatory insects, fungi, diseases, or animals (including humans). They can also be used to attract other species. Bees, for instance, are drawn to sweet-smelling flowers or sweet-tasting parts of a plant in order to spread pollen. Fruits attract animals who eat them, walk away, and eventually poop out the seeds, spreading the parent plant's progeny. It makes sense, then, that most flowers—like rose petals, violets, and nasturtiums—are low in toxins. So are most fruits—but sometimes only when the seeds are mature. For example, the common wild persimmon (*Diospyros virginiana*) native to North America produces one of my favorite fruits. When ripe, it's as luscious and sensual as a perfectly ripe apricot with the slightest hint of honey; when immature, its intense astringency will leave you gasping. (Captain John Smith, who established the first permanent English settlement in the New World at Jamestown, Virginia, in 1607, learned this the hard way when he tried this exotic fruit of a strange, unknown land and noted, "If it is not ripe it will draw a man's mouth awrie with much torment.") This is the persimmon tree's way of using allelochemicals to discourage animals from eating its fruit until the seeds are ready to be dispersed. Allelochemicals are even present in underground parts of plants, such as roots, corms, tubers, and rhizomes. The chemicals that conifer trees produce in their roots to repel other plants vary depending on the size and type of threat the tree detects from an intruding neighbor. And despite what we have been told about how leaving the skin on a potato is a healthy choice, the skin is actually the most toxic part of this staple food. Acting as the barrier between potential external threats and the potato, the skin is where the plant's toxins do their job to ward off fungi, pests, insects, and other predators.

So, what happens when a plant's natural defenses are removed or minimized? The domesticated plants we find in our grocery stores that look so fresh and healthy have been genetically modified through a number of techniques—from artificial selection to radiation—to make them larger, sweeter, easier to harvest, more productive, easier to ship, and more available year-round. Many of these processes invariably reduce the plants' toxins, essentially stripping them of their natural defenses to fend off diseases, insects, fungi, and even hostile takeovers by invasive plant species. We are left with defenseless plants that we in turn must bombard with herbicides, fungicides, and pesticides to protect them—adding those pollutants to our air, our water, and ourselves. And, I would argue, we're left defenseless as consumers as well. Although the toxins in these plants have been reduced, they haven't been eliminated. Yet we're told that to eat them year-round, even daily, is the healthiest choice we can make. Our lack of awareness about plants' native toxicity—and our rejection of eating vegetables only when they are in season—mean that we are, essentially, slowly poisoning ourselves. This is especially problematic for plants containing toxins such as oxalates, which can build up in our bodies over time.

Even worse, through domestication and genetic manipulation, we've also reduced these plants' nutritional density, medicinal value, and flavor. The produce in our grocery stores is far less nutritious than its predecessors of even a few decades ago. According to a 2007 report by the Organic Center—spurred by a symposium at the American Association for the Advancement of Science—American agriculture's unwavering emphasis on increasing crop yields has resulted in a steady decline in crops' nutritional value. The report notes, "As breeders have programmed plants to produce larger tomatoes, shorter-statured wheat with bigger grain heads, and corn that can tolerate closer spacing in the field, these plants have devoted less energy to other factors, like sinking deep roots and generating health-promoting compounds known as phytochemicals, many of which are antioxidants and vitamins." In corn and wheat plants, higher yields have correlated to falling levels of protein (a 0.3 percent decline in every decade of the 20th century) and rising levels of starch (an increase of the same amount, 0.3 percent, over the same time period). The report notes that a team of US Department of Agriculture researchers found that in 14 varieties of wheat grown between 1873 and 2000, when the average per-acre harvest more than tripled, the wheat's micronutrient content declined dramatically—for example, 28 percent less iron, 34 percent less zinc, and 36 percent less selenium over that period. Higher tomato yields correlate with lower vitamin C and lycopene, while cows produce more milk that's less concentrated with fat and protein.

In *Eating on the Wild Side: The Missing Link to Optimum Health,* Jo Robinson notes that the kernels of modern corn's ancestor, called teosinte, were 30 percent protein and 2 percent sugar. Compare this to contemporary varieties that are as high as 40 percent sugar. Robinson has noted that "eating corn this sweet can have the same impact on blood sugar as eating a Snickers candy bar or doughnut." When Robinson compared six wild varieties of apples to six modern varieties, she found that the wild varieties had *475 times* more phytonutrients. The Ginger Gold, a relatively new apple, has so few phytonutrients that it fails to even register on the scale. Yet a purple potato native to Peru has 28 times more cancer-fighting anthocyanins than common russet potatoes. These realities are one reason to look for what are called heirloom varieties — earlier versions of fruit and vegetable plants that have not had so many nutrients domesticated out of them. Local growers often opt for these varieties because they are more nutritious and taste better, so farmer's markets are good places to look for them. Many garden and seed supply companies sell heirloom varieties that you can grow yourself.

Meanwhile, wild plants left unmolested frequently have greater nutritional value than their domesticated, monocrop counterparts. For instance, nutritional tests show that foraged wild dandelion has twice as much calcium and fiber and two and a half times as much iron as store-bought dandelion; wild dandelion also has seven times more phytonutrients than spinach, which we consider a "superfood." Mallow, a common "weed," has more calcium than milk and eight times as much iron as spinach by volume. In fact, according to plant forager John Kallas, who wrote *Edible Wild Plants,* wild leafy food sources account for four of the top five leafy sources of omega-3s and manganese, two of the top five leafy sources of vitamin A, and three of the top five leafy sources of copper. The top seven leafy sources of iron and zinc and the top five leafy sources of calcium are all wild. And the benefits extend to the whole spectrum of plants.

When you start to rethink wild plants as health-food powerhouses rather than noxious weeds, adding them to your diet begins to make sense. They're free, they're nutritious, and once your eyes begin to open to the possibilities, they are *everywhere*. For me, this awakening began when I was a youngster growing up in suburban New Jersey. I never went anywhere without my Peterson's *Field Guide to Edible Wild Plants,* and more than once I bounded into the kitchen with fistfuls of *Chenopodium berlandieri,* commonly called lamb's quarters or wild spinach, that I'd found growing along the chain-link fence at the local elementary school. I had no idea that archaeologists believe this may have been one of the first plants that East Coast Native Americans domesticated almost 7,000 years ago. Nor did I understand that it was far more nutrient-dense than any plant we could have bought at the grocery store. I was simply excited to have foraged fresh greens that I could cook for my family and was certain they'd share that excitement. Well, *no,* not necessarily. To them, as with so many families of the 1970s and '80s, my treasures were potentially lethal weeds of dubious provenance, clearly not the waxed, polished, cleaned, wrapped, and sell-by-dated "fresh" vegetables that earned the USDA seal of approval.

Despite my family's lukewarm reaction to this first foraging, I never quit. I was like a birder with a life list. To keep track, I would save a leaf from each plant I positively identified or harvested for the first time and press it into the corresponding page in my Peterson's guide. Pretty soon my small field guide was bursting. Still, no matter how many plants I correctly identified, there always seemed to be others, supposedly right in my neck of the woods. Where were they? I figured they must be only in remote, pristine areas. That is, until I went to Central Park in New York City.

It was 2002, and I had convinced Christina, my wife of just two years, to come with me on a foraging tour led by legendary urban forager "Wildman" Steve Brill. (By now, Christina was starting to realize that there was no simple "walk in the woods" or "walk through the park" with me.) Brill had been conducting underground (aka illegal) foraging tours in Central Park until the authorities busted him in an undercover sting operation in 1986. His arrest was picked up by media outlets around the country, and the response was so strongly in his favor that the park eventually hired him to run his tours. But the relationship did not last, and he reverted to his underground tours. Even then, I was starting to feel that foraging was a simple, powerful way to protest a system — controlled by multinational food corporations based on monocropping — that was increasingly disconnecting people from their food and environment. Brill exemplified this form of protest, and I had long wanted to take one of his courses.

We met the Wildman and the rest of the participants at the entrance to Central Park, across the street from the American Museum of Natural History. Dressed for a safari — from his khaki-colored clothes to his Livingstone-style hat — Brill looked the part of a man who would lead us in search of elusive, renegade plants deep in whatever wilds still existed in a place that saw 38 million visitors a year. He collected $10 from each of us and removed his rucksack to offer to sell copies of his book, *Identifying and Harvesting Edible and Medicinal Plants in Wild (and Not So Wild) Places,* and jeweler's loupes, handy for any plant identification requiring magnification. When all the transactions were finished, he said, "Follow me," turned around, and started walking away. I stared into the distance, trying to discern which patch of woods or thicket we were headed toward. But after only a few steps, Brill stopped and turned around.

"Look at your feet," he said. I obeyed. I saw grass.

"What do you see?" he asked. I still saw grass.

"Look closely," he said. "Really closely. What else do you see besides grass?"

As I scrutinized the earth in front of my feet, plants with leaves of varying shapes and sizes and shades of green began to appear before my eyes. And, as my mind began to loosen up, I slowly realized that some of these were the very plants that I'd long searched for — sheep sorrel, curly dock, broad leaf plantain, wood sorrel! When I returned home with my "new" eyes, I could see these plants growing in my own backyard and between sidewalk cracks. I didn't have to trek through wilderness to find them; they were hiding in plain sight. It was my first lesson that wild edible plants are accessible everywhere, as long as you know how to look for them.

And look for them you should. Foraging lets us source the highest-quality, most nutrient-dense plants possible while ensuring that we are eating hyper-seasonally, bonding with our environment, and observing the consequences of our actions. It's the very antithesis of walking into a grocery store and plucking a waxed Red Delicious apple or plastic bag of lettuce from a shelf. Instead, it requires all of your attention, research, and senses. Spotting a patch of ramps isn't as much about the vein structure in the leaves as it is about a subtle yet unmistakable shade of green that can easily be seen from a distance. The scent of American basswood flowers in bloom or the leaves of the spicebush can confirm an identification without even seeing the plants themselves. The degree of bitterness in an acorn will hint at the variety of tree and help you decide whether it's worth your time and effort to collect.

The crispness in the air, dampness on the ground, or position of the sun can also tip you off to the plants you should be looking for and how you should look for them. The sound of a nearby stream, the roar of traffic on a highway, children's laughter at a park, or silence in the middle of the woods all help you determine how land is being used, and whether it's safe for foraging; for instance, you wouldn't want to forage plants in a park where pesticides have been applied, or beside a busy roadway.

Our backyards, our walk to work or around town, and even our jogging trails all offer opportunities to routinely observe and harvest plants. Traditional hunter-gatherers don't "go foraging" or "go hunting"; instead, they forage and hunt all the time as part of their daily lives. They're always on the lookout for food, and they take advantage of any opportunity to identify new sources of food, check on known food sources as they change and mature throughout the year, and procure food whenever possible. I matured the most as a forager the year we rented a house in Frenchtown, New Jersey, a couple of blocks from the Delaware River. I ran the same three-mile stretch of riverside year-round and watched as plants progressed through their life cycles and changed through the seasons. Over that year I formed relationships with these plants—such as bee balm, mayapple, poke, and wild bergamot—and learned a great deal about them, information I still use today. Certainly, setting aside dedicated time to focus exclusively on identifying and collecting wild plants is worthwhile, but being attentive to foraging as part of our daily existence should embed this practice in our lives and yield the best results.

Once you are more knowledgeably sourcing plants, the next step is to learn how to process them safely to gain the most nutrition. Here, we can again look to the past. Before the Agricultural Revolution (around 15,000 years ago), our ancestors had to forage for every vegetable and fruit. Not only were they up against the biological barriers I described in Chapter 1 — that is, humans are not built to digest plants — but they also had to figure out how to make plants safe to consume. Through trial and error, they learned to cook or process plants to detoxify them enough to access their nutrition. Once they made stone tools, about 3.3 million years ago, some wild tubers, corms, and rhizomes — the prehistoric equivalent of today's root vegetables — could be detoxified through slicing and dehydrating. Foods like acorns could be rendered safe through submersion in water, which leaches out their toxic, water-soluble tannins. Heat-sensitive toxins in other nutrient-rich root vegetables could be minimized through baking in underground earth ovens. A fairly recent example of this technology was used by Native Americans of the Eastern Seaboard who harvested arrow arum (*Peltandra virginica*) as a staple food. This thick, starchy, and abundant rhizome contains raphides, bundles of calcium oxalate needles. When ingested, they pierce the skin and release a protease compound that causes the lips, mouth, and throat to burn and swell — ultimately enough to kill you by closing off your windpipe. To avoid this, Native Americans dug pits into which they would place the arrow arum rhizomes, covering them with soil and building fires on top to bake the roots for as long as 24 hours. Heating the roots didn't eliminate the protease toxin, but it did disable the raphides so that the toxin couldn't be delivered into the skin's soft tissues. Thus, they could gain all the benefits of the plant's starches while neutralizing its dangers. Another good example of a toxin-bypassing technology is geophagy, which we'll discuss at length in Chapter 8 when I take you to Bolivia. There, Aymara Indians of the Altiplano region of the Andes still safely consume highly toxic native potatoes by eating them with clay. The clay binds with the toxin, transforming it so that the body doesn't absorb it but instead simply passes it harmlessly through the digestive tract.

These are excellent technologies for making plants safe and digestible, but the easiest and most obvious way to detoxify many plants is through a natural process that our ancestors learned was happening all around them: fermentation. Simply put, fermentation is the transformation of plants (and other foods and substances) by bacteria, yeasts, and other microorganisms that exist in the air, on our food, in our soil—in short, everywhere. In the most basic sense, fermentation works with environmental processes instead of against them. If you're not too squeamish, you can think of it as "controlled rot," where we are controlling temperature, oxygen, salt, hydration, time, and other factors to physically transform raw materials into their safest, most nutrient-dense and bioavailable forms. Through a combination of chemical and physical processes, fermentation can reduce or deactivate a range of chemical compounds. Our ancestors could have used it to detoxify roots, tubers, and rhizomes by doing something as simple as burying them in the anaerobic environment of a marsh and pulling them out weeks later.

We eat fermented foods all the time. Sauerkraut, beer, yogurt, and pickles are familiar to most of us, but increasingly more exotic examples are coming to the fore, such as kombucha, miso, and kimchi. You will see the word *fermentation* throughout this book because it's a technology that can be used with a whole host of foods, including dairy (to make yogurt, kefir, and cheese), grains (to make bread such as sourdough), and meats (such as salami). In the case of a plant, like the cabbage in my recipe for Amazing Sauerkraut on page 50, it involves submerging the vegetable in a saltwater brine, an oxygen-free environment that creates the ideal conditions for the natural beneficial bacteria on the vegetable to do a variety of work. This includes feeding off the sugars and starches in the vegetable and producing probiotics as well as lactic acid—which in this case is helpful, because the drop in pH that accompanies the production of lactic acid creates an extremely safe environment and lets you easily and safely store the vegetable for a long time. (Probiotics, which we return to repeatedly in this book, are beneficial microorganisms such as bacteria and yeasts that exist in and on our bodies and perform a multitude of functions relating to health. Certain foods, and certain methods of processing, can introduce more probiotics into our systems.) Furthermore, remember the concept of how technologies enabled our ancestors to do outside our bodies what some animals are biologically built to do inside theirs, such as cows eating grass? Fermenting does this for us. It begins to predigest the food so that our digestive tract doesn't have to work as hard, and it also makes nutrients accessible to our bodies that otherwise wouldn't be.

Few things I will talk about in this book offer a more immediate, easy, fun, and fulfilling way to reestablish a healthy, ancestral relationship with food than the simple acts of seasonal foraging and employing the technology of fermentation. By becoming contemporary gatherers and using modern versions of the same technologies our ancestors discovered, we can circumvent a process that is stripping our plants of their nutrition while falsely presenting these foods as healthy choices. You might not have the time — or the comfort level — to forage for an entire meal. So, start small. Find a patch of wild spinach (maybe it will even be by the fence next to your kid's elementary school) and bring home a handful or two. Wash the leaves, dry them, and add them to your store-bought salad for dinner. Rather than serving that genetically modified, out-of-season asparagus that magically turns up in the grocery store in late November, consider a local autumn vegetable, such as cabbage or carrots, that you have fermented in a salt brine to maximize its nutrition and longevity, as well as a flavor that conveys a powerful sense of terroir. Even these small steps represent the beginning of a sea change in regaining control over your food and learning how to eat like a human.

FORAGING TIPS AND RECIPES

FIRST STEPS TO FORAGING

How to start foraging? First, educate yourself. Foraging has been growing more popular and mainstream in the last several years, and there are so many information sources, including foraging tours, books, apps, and Facebook groups, that it can actually be a little overwhelming. So, I'd suggest some basics:

1. Consider taking a foraging tour where you live. The Association of Foragers is a great source: foragers-association.org.

2. Gather a variety of books on the subject and dig deeply into them. You already know two of my favorites — Peterson's *Field Guide to Edible Wild Plants* and Steve Brill's *Identifying and Harvesting Edible and Medicinal Plants in Wild (and Not So Wild) Places* — but here's a short list of my other go-to references:
   - *Edible Wild Plants: Wild Foods from Dirt to Plate* (The Wild Food Adventure Series, Book 1) by John Kallas
   - *The New Wildcrafted Cuisine: Exploring the Exotic Gastronomy of Local Terroir* by Pascal Baudar
   - *The Forager's Harvest: A Guide to Identifying, Harvesting, and Preparing Edible Wild Plants* by Samuel Thayer
   - *Shoots and Greens of Early Spring in Northeastern North America* by Steve Brill

3. Put together a foraging kit. Here's what's in mine; it fits easily into a small backpack and I keep it with me at all times:
   - Reference guides. Titles vary depending on specific circumstances and seasons, but I typically carry at least three, and I suggest that you identify a plant using all three guides before eating it.
   - Collection vessels. Avoid plastic bags because they cause the plants to sweat, especially when it's hot. I use brown paper lunch bags. They are a good size, reusable, and breathable, and they fold flat to fit in my back pocket.
   - A pocketknife. I always carry a pocketknife. *Always.*
   - A digging stick, ubiquitous in traditional societies around the world. These are usually nothing more than a medium-size stick with a sharpened end to break up the soil and extract roots like tubers and rhizomes. Find or make one

about 14 inches long and about 1½ inches in diameter; tie a string around one end so it can hang from your wrist when not in use.

The Wild Top Five

Here's a list of the top five wild greens that you should be able to find in your own backyard or in a nearby park. I like these because they are ubiquitous, safe, easy to identify, and easy to cook with. Do not forage in an area that has been chemically sprayed, and make sure to properly identify any new plant in at least three different sources (see references above). You can use these greens in the recipes that follow, among others:

1. Dandelion (spring, late summer)
2. Garlic mustard (spring, summer, early fall)
3. Wild spinach, aka lamb's quarters (spring, summer)
4. Purslane (spring, summer, fall)
5. Chickweed (spring, summer, fall)

WILD GREENS, ROASTED BONE MARROW, AND SOURDOUGH

SERVES 4

Many wild plants are slightly bitter, and the best way to cut the bitterness is with fat. That is why dandelion greens are often cooked with bacon grease. High-quality butter, lard, and bone marrow are also excellent options. This recipe is one of my favorite ways of using fat to cut the bitterness of wild greens. It is an adaptation of Fergus Henderson's roasted marrow bones, a popular dish from his London restaurant, St. John.

6 (3-inch-long) marrow bones (ask the butcher for center-cut bones)
Lard or other fat, for greasing
3 cups slightly bitter wild greens (such as dandelion leaves or arugula)
1 tablespoon finely chopped wild field garlic, shallot, or garlic
2 teaspoons capers, rinsed and chopped
2 tablespoons extra virgin olive oil
2 teaspoons freshly squeezed lemon juice
Kosher salt and freshly ground black pepper
6 slices Airfield Sourdough Bread (page 135), toasted

Preheat the oven to 450°F.

Stand the marrow bones in a lightly greased roasting pan and roast for 15 to 25 minutes, until the marrow has puffed slightly and is warm in the center.

While the bones are roasting, combine the greens, garlic, and capers in a medium bowl. In a small bowl or jar, whisk together the oil and lemon juice, then season very lightly with salt and very generously with pepper. Toss the salad with the dressing.

To serve, stand the bones on a platter, sprinkle with salt, and arrange the dressed salad around the bones. To eat, use a marrow spoon specially designed for the task, or simply use the handle of a regular spoon to extract the warm marrow from the center of each bone and spread it on the sourdough toasts. Add another sprinkle of salt and top it with some of the dressed salad.

WILD SPRING FRITTATA

SERVES 4 TO 6

Milder wild greens such as lamb's quarters, violets, and mallow lend themselves well to sautéing for use in frittatas, quiches, and other egg dishes. This frittata recipe is my family's go-to on a busy night when we need a quick, delicious, and nourishing dish.

> 4 tablespoons butter, lard, tallow, or bacon grease, divided
> 3 cups assorted wild greens, chopped
> 12 large eggs
> ½ cup heavy cream
> Sea salt and freshly ground black pepper
> 1 cup shredded cheese (such as Gruyère, fontina, or cheddar)

Preheat the oven to 350°F with a rack in the middle.

In a large cast-iron skillet, heat 2 tablespoons of the butter over medium heat. Add the greens and sauté until softened, about 5 minutes. Set aside to cool slightly.

In a large bowl, whisk the eggs until blended. Add the cream, season with salt and pepper, and whisk until blended. Stir in the greens and shredded cheese.

Place the same cast-iron skillet over medium-high heat and add the remaining 2 tablespoons butter. Once the skillet is hot and the butter has melted, slowly pour in the egg mixture. Cook for a few minutes to set the bottom, then transfer to the oven. Bake for 35 to 40 minutes, until the eggs are set but not overcooked.

Let the frittata rest for a few minutes, then invert the skillet over a cutting board or platter and cut into wedges.

WILD PESTO

Pesto is an excellent way to make use of two different flavors that come from certain wild greens. For a traditional-flavored pesto, use garlic mustard leaves—they possess a flavor perfectly described by their name, that of both garlic and mustard greens. Or, for a refreshing, lighter pesto, use the lemony sheep sorrel or wood sorrel. Pesto is incredibly versatile. It pairs well with tomatoes and fresh Mozzarella (page 192) and can be used as a dip or spread, a base layer on a Sourdough Pizza Crust (page 144), and a topping for grilled meats, such as Grilled Chicken Hearts with Wild Pesto (page 83).

> 1½ cups sheep sorrel, wood sorrel, and/or garlic mustard leaves
> ½ cup grated Parmesan cheese
> ½ cup extra virgin olive oil
> 3 garlic cloves, peeled, or 1 tablespoon minced field garlic or wild onion
> ½ cup toasted black walnuts or sunflower seeds

Put all the ingredients in a food processor and pulse several times, until they're coarsely chopped. Scrape down the work bowl, then process continuously until the sauce is smooth. Use immediately or store in a tightly sealed container in the refrigerator for up to 1 week or in the freezer for several months.

HOW I LEARNED TO STOP WORRYING
AND LOVE POKE

Poke is an excellent example of a widely available toxic plant that can be easily detoxified in your kitchen. Unfortunately, most recipes are overly cautious and instruct you to boil it much longer than needed. This results in a lifeless, mushy, greenish-gray mass that, along with its toxins, has lost much of its nutrition, flavor, and texture. My good friend and master forager, Steve Adams, has developed the following detoxification strategy that ensures the final product is not only safe but also colorful, vibrant, and delicious.

12 poke shoots and leaves (harvested in the early spring when
they are no more than 8 to 10 inches tall)

Wash the poke shoots and leaves by submerging them in a bowl of water and agitating them to dislodge any dirt, grit, or debris. Let them sit for a couple of minutes for the debris to settle. Lift out the poke, discard the water, and repeat until the shoots and leaves are clean. Cut the poke into 1½-inch pieces. This increases the surface area and exposes the ends of the plant's vascular tissues.

You'll need one pot large enough to hold the raw poke along with enough water to completely cover it without crowding, and a second pot that's twice as large as the first.

Fill the larger pot with water (see note below) and bring to a rapid boil; leave it boiling. Meanwhile, fill a large bowl with a combination of water and ice. Put a colander in the sink.

Put the sliced poke in the smaller pot and cover with cold water. Cover the pot and bring to a boil over high heat. As soon as the water begins to boil, set a timer for 1 minute.

At the end of 1 minute, drain the poke in the colander (the water will be pink and should be discarded), return the poke to the pot, and immediately cover it with water from the already boiling pot. Resume the full boil and boil the poke for 1 minute without covering. Drain in the colander and discard the water, which will be much less pink than the first batch.

Return the poke to the pot and cover with more boiling water, and resume the full boil again, uncovered. Once boiling, reduce the heat to a simmer and cook for 2 minutes.

Using a slotted spoon, transfer the poke to the ice-water bath to halt the cooking process. Once it's cooled to your liking, you can eat it immediately, use it in a variety of dishes such as Poke Sallet (page 44), or refrigerate or freeze for longer-term storage. When detoxified, poke has an appearance, texture, and flavor similar to that of asparagus and can be used in very similar ways.

Note:

As an alternative to plain water, add chunks of ginger, fresh herbs, and onion skins and trimmings and let them simmer enough to flavor the water, lending a complementary character to the cooked poke. Discard this flavored water and the solids at the end of the detoxification process, as they will have absorbed the toxins leached from the poke.

POKE SALLET

Sallet is a medieval word that simply means "cooked greens." Poke sallet is a traditional southern dish that takes slightly different forms depending on the region, but in almost all cases, the detoxified poke shoots and greens are sautéed in bacon grease and finished with apple cider vinegar. Sometimes eggs are added, and that is how I like to make it because of the high-quality nutrition the eggs add to the dish.

6 large eggs
1 pound bacon, chopped
1 large onion, diced
2 garlic cloves, minced
2 cups detoxified poke shoots and leaves (see page 42)
Sea salt and freshly ground black pepper
Apple cider vinegar

In a medium bowl, whisk the eggs until fully blended.

Cook the bacon in a sauté pan over medium heat until crisp. Using a slotted spoon, transfer it to a plate lined with paper towels to drain. Add the onion to the hot fat and cook until translucent, about 5 minutes. Add the garlic and cook for a few minutes to soften.

Increase the heat to medium-high, add the poke, and cook for about 5 minutes, until warmed through and any liquid released from the greens has evaporated. Add the eggs and stir to scramble until cooked through. Serve finished with a little salt, pepper, and apple cider vinegar to taste.

ACORN FLOUR

MAKES ABOUT 3 CUPS

Acorns are easy to find, identify, and detoxify. They were used extensively prehistorically around the world and are still in use in some places, such as Korea. Fortunately, the primary toxin in acorns, tannic acid, is water-soluble, so acorns can be made safe to eat by soaking in water. Many foraging guides advocate extensive processing of whole acorns in repeated changes of boiling water. But by crushing the acorns first, you can use cold water to accomplish the same goal faster and with better results. Crushing increases the surface area and makes the leaching process more effective.

Acorn flour can be used in a variety of dishes and can be combined with wheat flour in just about any baked goods recipe, from pancakes to bread. Simply substitute acorn flour for some of the wheat flour to add nutrition, flavor, and texture while also reducing the amount of gluten and carbohydrates in the recipe. I've had great results when substituting between 20 and 50 percent of wheat flour with acorn flour.

2 pounds acorns (about 1 gallon, if using a gallon-size bucket)

Using a rock, hammer, or nutcrackers, gently crack the acorns' shells and remove the nut meat inside. Discard the shells. Peel off and discard as much of the brown "skin" adhering to the nuts as possible. Put the shelled acorns in a blender or food processor, add enough water to completely submerge the acorns, and process into a fine slurry. This increases the surface area and allows fast and efficient leaching.

Acorn flour was traditionally leached in streams, where the moving water would carry the leached tannins away from the acorns. That process can be replicated in a sink using a constant stream of water from the faucet in about 20 minutes (Method 1) or, if you are concerned about water consumption, in a large glass container over the course of a few days (Method

2). Note that different varieties of acorns contain varied amounts of tannic acid and therefore require different processing times. For example, acorns from white oaks have very little tannic acid and don't need much process-ing, while acorns from black oaks and red oaks have higher tannic acid levels and thus require more time to fully detoxify.

Method 1: Line a colander with a cheesecloth, tea towel, or T-shirt and put it in the sink. Slowly pour the blender contents into it. Gather the oppo-site corners of the cloth together and tie them to make a makeshift bag. Lift the bag from the colander and place the knotted ends on top of a faucet, hanging the bag so that the surface of the acorn flour is resting a couple of inches below the faucet opening. Slowly turn the faucet on cold and adjust the flow so that the water streaming into the acorn flour matches the stream pouring from the bottom. This will prevent an overflow of water and acorn flour while ensuring the leaching process happens as quickly as possible.

Allow the crushed acorns to leach for about 20 minutes, then taste a small amount to determine if there is any tannic acid left. Tannic acid tastes bitter and astringent. The acorns should taste bland and slightly earthy. If you detect any tannic acid, continue the process, checking every 10 minutes or so.

Method 2: Pour the blender contents into a large glass jar. The jar should be large enough that the ground acorns do not fill it more than halfway; if necessary, use multiple jars. Fill the jar with cold tap water, stir, and cover. Place the jar in the refrigerator overnight. The water will turn brown, indicating that the tannic acid is leaching from the acorns. The next day, remove the lid and slowly tip the jar to carefully pour off as much water as possible while keeping the ground acorns in the jar. Refill with clean water, stir, cover, and return to the refrigerator. Repeat every 24 hours until the water no longer changes color.

Line a colander with a cheesecloth, tea towel, or T-shirt and slowly pour the water and ground acorns through to drain. Taste a small amount to determine if there is any tannic acid left. Tannic acid tastes bitter and astringent. The acorns should taste bland and slightly earthy. If you detect any tannic acid, return the ground acorns to the jar, fill with water, and repeat the process.

Drying Acorn Flour

Once the acorn flour is sufficiently detoxified, squeeze the cloth containing the ground acorns to remove as much moisture as possible. Spread the ground acorns on a rimmed baking sheet and dehydrate in your oven at its lowest setting (for most of us that is 170°F) for several hours, until completely dry. If necessary, process the dried acorn meal in a blender or food processor until the desired consistency is reached. Use immediately or store in an airtight container for up to 2 years.

FERMENTATION TIPS AND RECIPES

FERMENTATION VESSELS

Before you start fermenting plants, it's important to choose the right vessel. In the process of fermenting, vegetables produce lactic acid, and most metals—especially aluminum—do not do well in the presence of acid. You can use high-quality stainless steel, however, since it doesn't react negatively to acidic environments. Plastic, because it is soft and easy to scratch, is undesirable, because it provides places for unsafe pathogens to live. Chemicals in the plastic can also leach into your food.

Vessels made out of glass and ceramic are ideal options. Glass mason jars and ceramic crocks make fantastic fermentation vessels. Mason jars are readily available at most grocery and hardware stores. Stay away from older glass containers, though, because some may contain lead, which can leach into your food. Fermentation crocks are more difficult to find on store shelves and are expensive to ship because of their size and weight. Check with your local hardware store; many makers of these crocks will ship them directly to the store at no extra cost. Avoid old ceramic crocks, because they often contain invisible cracks that can harbor unsafe bacteria as well as allow liquids to leak onto your counter.

FERMENTATION WEIGHTS

Fermenting vegetables is an anaerobic activity, which means it takes place in the absence of oxygen. The oxygen-free environment is created by submerging the vegetables in brine (a mixture of water and salt). Unfortunately, many vegetables want to float and need to be weighted down to keep them submerged. There are a variety of ways to keep them below the surface of the brine during the fermentation process:

- Pack the jar incredibly tight with vegetables so they are forced to stay submerged. This works well with large pieces of vegetables, such as carrots, but will not work with finely chopped or shredded vegetables, such as cabbage for sauerkraut.
- Use a commercial weight designed for the purpose. Look online to find all sorts of glass, ceramic, stainless steel, and even wooden weights and contraptions of different sizes specially designed for mason jars and ceramic crocks.
- Use rocks from your yard of the proper size. Wash the rocks well with soap and water, then completely submerge them in boiling water for at least 5 minutes before you use them for the first time.
- Use your fingers! Several times a day simply push the contents of the jar below the surface of the brine with clean hands. While tedious, this lets you interact with your ferment, observe how it changes, and, if you lick your fingers each time, get a sense of how the flavor changes.

FERMENTATION COVERS

It's a good idea to cover your fermentation vessel to keep bugs, dust, and other contaminants out. Good options include:

- A kitchen towel or paper towel secured with a rubber band.
- A plastic mason jar lid. Aluminum lids that come with mason jars will corrode in the presence of the acid and salt. These

inexpensive plastic versions work better, although you should not screw them on tightly.

* Commercially designed covers for mason jars with airlocks. These airlocks release oxygen as it is replaced by the heavier carbon dioxide to help create an anaerobic environment even above the surface of the brine.

DIGITAL KITCHEN SCALE

This is one of the most important tools in my kitchen; it will be needed for most of the recipes in this book. You can find an inexpensive, reliable scale online.

AMAZING SAUERKRAUT

Makes about 1 gallon

If your idea of sauerkraut is that mouth-puckering, rather slimy stuff that's piled on top of your hot dog, think again. Sauerkraut can be made from nothing more than cabbage and salt, but the addition of sour green apples, onions, and spices elevates it to something amazing.

> 2 heads cabbage (green and/or red)
> 1 sour apple, peeled if desired, cored, and thinly sliced
> ½ onion, thinly sliced
> 1 bay leaf
> ⅛ to ¼ teaspoon caraway seeds
> 2 or 3 juniper berries
> Sea salt

Equipment Needed

> Kitchen scale
> 4 (1-quart) mason jars, 2 (2-quart) mason jars, or 1 gallon-size
>   ceramic crock
> Plastic lid(s) or cloth cover(s) (see page 48)
> Fermentation weight(s) (see page 48)

Remove the outermost leaves of the cabbage. Set aside some of the larger leaves to cover and submerge the cabbage during fermentation. Wash the remaining cabbage, cutting out any bruised sections, and remove the core. Use a knife or food processor to shred the cabbage.

Place a large bowl on the scale and press the tare button to set to zero. Transfer the shredded cabbage to the bowl, then add the apple, onion, bay leaf, caraway seeds, and juniper berries. Take the weight of all the ingredients and multiply by 0.02 to calculate the amount of salt you will need.

For instance, if your vegetable mixture weighs 1,000 grams, you will need 20 grams of salt.

Add the salt to the bowl and mix and massage it thoroughly into the cabbage. This physical action will help the salt draw out the moisture required to submerge the ferment under the brine.

Transfer this mixture, including the liquid, to your fermentation vessel(s) a bit at a time and pack it tightly. Continue to pack in the vegetables until they come no higher than within 2 inches of the top of each vessel. Do not overfill, as the contents will expand during fermentation, and you must leave room for the weight. The liquid released from the cabbage must cover the weight while still leaving 1 inch of air space at the top.

Place the reserved large leaves over the shredded vegetable mixture to help keep it submerged, then add your fermentation weight. If there is not enough liquid to completely submerge the vegetables, prepare a 2 percent brine (made by mixing water and salt at the same 2 percent rate as above), and pour it in until you have enough liquid.

Cover the vessel loosely with a lid or cloth and place it in a basement, closet, or pantry—the ideal fermentation temperature is 62°F. By the end of the first week, the fermentation process will have begun, visible by the production of gas bubbles. At this point, taste a piece of cabbage daily, and always make sure it stays completely submerged. If mold appears on the surface of the brine, carefully remove with a spoon and discard. When the sauerkraut has reached your preferred flavor and texture, cover the vessel tightly and move it to the refrigerator, where it will keep for up to 6 months. If you fermented in a large crock, you can repack the sauerkraut in mason jars for cold storage. I find that fermenting for 10 days is ideal for both flavor and texture, but you can let it ferment for up to several weeks.

FERMENTED CARROT STICKS

MAKES ABOUT 1 QUART

These are a great addition to the kids' lunch boxes. I like to initiate the fermentation on Friday to begin to use them in lunches on Monday. The flavors continue to develop over the next few days, and by Wednesday I stick the jar in the fridge. Making these takes only a few minutes longer than simply cutting carrot sticks for lunches but delivers much more flavor and nutrition—plus loads of probiotics.

> 3 to 6 large carrots
> Sea salt

Equipment Needed

> Kitchen scale
> 1 (1-quart) mason jar
> Plastic lid or cloth cover (see page 48)

Peel and trim the carrots. (Reserve the peels and ends for making Trash Bone Broth, page 79.) Cut the carrots into approximately 4-inch-long sections, then cut lengthwise into quarters.

Place the empty mason jar on the scale. Press the tare button on the scale to set to zero. Neatly stand the carrot sticks in the jar, making sure you have enough pieces so that they fit as tightly as possible. This will ensure that they remain in place below the brine without the use of a weight. Pour in enough water to cover the carrot sticks, but leave approximately 1 inch of space between the top of the water and the top of the jar. Record the weight. Multiply the weight by 0.02 to calculate the amount of salt you will need. For instance, if your vegetable mixture weighs 1,000 grams, you will need 20 grams of salt.

Pour the water from the jar into a medium bowl, add the calculated amount of salt to the water, and mix until thoroughly dissolved. Pour the brine back into the jar to cover the carrots.

Cover loosely with a plastic lid by not screwing it on completely, or with a paper towel secured with a rubber band, and place the vessel in a basement, closet, or pantry to ferment — the ideal fermentation temperature is 62°F. The carrots are full of sugar and will usually begin to ferment within 2 to 3 days, visible by the production of gas bubbles. At this point, taste a carrot. Continue to ferment until the desired flavor and texture are achieved, then move the carrots to the fridge, where they will keep for up to 3 months. I usually ferment carrots for 3 to 5 days.

FERMENTED ROASTED RED PEPPERS

MAKES ABOUT 1 QUART

My family loves roasted red peppers. We eat them on pizza, in sandwiches, and as a base for sauces, so we like to make a large batch at a time. By fermenting them, we increase their flavor, shelf life, and nutrition. Plus, they are chock-full of probiotics.

6 red bell peppers
4 to 6 garlic cloves, peeled
3 fresh rosemary sprigs
3 fresh thyme sprigs
Sea salt

Equipment Needed

Kitchen scale
1 (1-quart) mason jar
Fermentation weight (see page 48)
Plastic lid or cloth cover (see page 48)

Preheat the oven to 400°F with a rack in the upper third.

Place the red peppers on their side on a rimmed baking sheet and roast until the top surface of the pepper is charred, about 20 minutes. Using tongs, turn the peppers and continue to roast and turn for another 20 minutes or so, until all their skins are charred, bubbly, and pulling away from the flesh. Transfer the roasted peppers to a bowl and cover with a plate. Allow the hot peppers to steam and cool for approximately 30 minutes.

Once the peppers are cool enough to handle, remove the stems and pull the charred skin away from the flesh. Slice the peppers in half and scrape out the seeds and ribs. Put the skinned and seeded roasted peppers in a bowl, along with any accumulated liquid.

Place the empty mason jar on the scale. Press the tare button on the scale to set to zero. Fill the jar with the roasted peppers and their liquid, garlic cloves, and rosemary and thyme sprigs. Fill the jar with water until the peppers are completely submerged, and record the weight. Multiply the weight by 0.02 to calculate the amount of salt you will need. For instance, if the combined weight of your peppers, herbs, and water is 1,000 grams, you will need 20 grams of salt.

Pour the liquid from the jar into a medium bowl, add the calculated amount of salt to the water, and mix until thoroughly dissolved. Pour the brine back into the jar to cover the contents.

Place a fermentation weight on top of the peppers to keep them submerged. Cover loosely with a plastic lid by not screwing down completely, or with a paper towel secured by a rubber band, and place the vessel in a basement, closet, or pantry to ferment—the ideal fermentation temperature is 62°F. After 5 to 7 days, the fermentation process will have begun, visible by the production of gas bubbles. At this point, cover the jar tightly and transfer to the refrigerator, where the peppers will keep for up to 6 months.

LACTO-CHIPS AND LACTO-FRIES

SERVES 4 TO 6

Imagine healthy potato chips or French fries . . . well, here they are. While conducting research in Peru on how the Quechua detoxify potatoes, I learned to make tocosh, a fermented potato food that is a staple in their traditional diet. The Quechua ferment whole potatoes in underground pits for months to detoxify them. The following recipe uses a variation on this process that shortens fermentation time by peeling and cutting the potatoes into fries or slicing them into chips. This increases the surface area while decreasing mass, helping the effects of the fermentation penetrate more quickly. Here's how this process makes potatoes a safer, healthier, more nutritious food:

1. Peeling the potatoes drastically reduces toxins.
2. Fermenting continues to lower the toxins and enhance digestibility.
3. Fermenting provides a pleasant sour flavor reminiscent of salt and vinegar chips.
4. Fermenting reduces the carbohydrates, making it a lower-glycemic food.
5. Reducing the carbohydrates through fermentation also diminishes the Maillard reaction; this is what happens when the sugars come in contact with high heat, producing browning on chips and fries. This is important because the Maillard reaction in these foods can produce dangerous carcinogenic acrylamides.

Simply by including a fermentation step and frying in high-quality animal fat, we can transform an unhealthy junk food into a safe and nourishing food that I am proud to feed my family. While this is a somewhat labor-intensive process, it's well worth it. When you make the fries, make a double batch and freeze half so you can grab a handful from the freezer and throw them directly into the deep fryer for an easy, last-minute side.

For the Chips

½ cup sea salt, plus more for seasoning

3 pounds potatoes (such as russet and/or sweet potatoes)

2 quarts animal fat (such as lard or tallow)

Equipment Needed

Large glass or ceramic fermentation vessel

Plastic lid or cloth cover (see page 48)

Deep fryer or large, heavy pot and thermometer

To make the brine, pour 1 gallon water into a large fermentation container and add the salt. Stir to combine and dissolve the salt. Set the brine aside.

Fill a large bowl with water. Peel the potatoes. As soon as each potato is peeled, place it in the bowl of water so that it does not oxidize while you are peeling the rest. Once all of the potatoes are peeled, use a food processor, mandoline, or sharp knife to slice them to a thickness of $\frac{1}{16}$ to $\frac{1}{8}$ inch.

Put the sliced potatoes in the brine. Make sure the water level is no less than 1 inch from the top of the vessel so that it doesn't overflow during fermentation. Cover the container with a cloth or lid that is not screwed on too tightly and set aside at room temperature to ferment. Fermentation, visible by the production of bubbles, should begin in a day or two. I usually ferment for a total of 3 to 5 days, depending on the temperature (less time if warmer, more if cooler) and on the desired flavor.

Pour the animal fat into a deep fryer or large, heavy pot and heat to 300°F.

While the fat is heating, drain the potato slices in a colander and rinse thoroughly several times. Spread out the slices in a single layer on a cooling rack or dish towel so that the moisture evaporates from the surface. If necessary, blot the tops with a towel. It is important to remove as much moisture as possible from the surface of the potato slices to prevent splattering when frying.

Once the fat is at 300°F and the surfaces of the potato slices are relatively dry, deep-fry in batches for 5 to 7 minutes, until the desired crispiness is achieved. Do not expect them to brown as much as regular potato chips.

Transfer the chips to a wire rack, crumpled-up brown paper, or paper towels, immediately sprinkle with salt, and toss to distribute. The chips can be eaten as soon as they cool or stored in an airtight container at room temperature for up to 1 week.

For the Fries

> ½ cup sea salt, plus more for seasoning
> 3 pounds potatoes (such as russet and/or sweet potatoes)
> 2 quarts animal fat (such as lard or tallow)
> Omega-naise (page 88) or Fermented Ketchup (page 101),
>   for serving

Equipment Needed

> Large glass or ceramic fermentation vessel
> Plastic lid or cloth cover (see page 48)
> Deep fryer or large, heavy pot and thermometer

To make the brine, pour 1 gallon water into a large fermentation container and add the salt. Stir to combine and dissolve the salt. Set the brine aside.

Fill a large bowl with water. Peel the potatoes. As soon as each potato is peeled, place it in the bowl of water so that it does not oxidize while you are peeling the rest. Once all of the potatoes are peeled, use a sharp knife to cut them lengthwise into approximately ⅜-inch slices, then cut the slices into approximately ⅜-inch strips to create French fries.

Put the cut potatoes in the brine. Make sure the water level is no less than 1 inch from the top of the vessel so that it doesn't overflow during fermentation. Cover the container with a cloth or lid that is not screwed on too tightly and set aside at room temperature to ferment. Fermentation, visible by the production of bubbles, should begin in a day or two. I usually ferment for a total of 3 to 5 days depending on the temperature (less time if warmer, more if cooler) and on the desired flavor.

Pour the animal fat into a deep fryer or heavy-duty pot and heat to 325°F.

While the fat is heating, drain the potatoes in a colander and rinse thoroughly several times. Spread out the fries in a single layer on a cooling rack or dish towel so that the moisture evaporates from the surface. If necessary, blot the tops with a towel. It is important to remove as much moisture as possible from the surface of the potatoes to prevent splattering when frying.

The best French fries are cooked twice. The first time actually cooks the potatoes and the second crisps the outsides. Once the fat is at 325°F and the surfaces of the fries are relatively dry, deep-fry in batches for 5 minutes. Transfer the fries to a wire rack, crumpled-up brown paper, or paper towels to cool.

Make sure the fries cool thoroughly before moving to the next step. The cooling process initiates several chemical and physical changes that help make a crispier and tastier result. Once the fries are thoroughly cooled, they can be either cooked again to finish or frozen for storage. To freeze, spread out the fries in a single layer on a rimmed baking sheet so that they freeze separately. Once frozen, transfer them to a resealable bag or container. Whenever you want fries, you can pull out as many as you want and throw them directly into the fryer for the final cook.

For the second, final frying, bring the fat to 375°F. Deep-fry the potatoes in batches for 3 to 5 minutes, until the desired crispiness is achieved. Do not expect them to brown as much as regular French fries.

Transfer the fries to a wire rack, crumpled-up brown paper, or paper towels, immediately sprinkle with salt, and toss to distribute. Eat while still warm, with mayo or ketchup, if desired.

Chapter 3

ANIMALS

MORE ANIMAL, LESS MEAT

It was 40 degrees below zero, and a polar wind was howling like a banshee down the riverine ridges of the near-distant mountains, whipping across the open plain of the northern Mongolian steppe and pinching my face with its frigid fingers. The cold was a living thing, working its way through even my minimally exposed skin and into my bones. A mere 50 feet away, a comforting billow of smoke rose and then flew from the peak of the *ger*—what you might know as a yurt, or a portable, round tent. It looked awfully warm and appealing, this home to the Mongolian herder who was crouching before me. Beneath his busy hands, steam rose and spun away from the body of the yak he had just felled with a single well-placed sledge-hammer strike that dropped the huge animal like a stone. As soon as the yak had hit the frozen ground, the herder dropped the hammer, picked up his knife, and severed the massive animal's jugular. Nothing in the northern Mongolian steppe goes to waste—most certainly not this yak's blood—and the herder caught every last drop in a metal pot before the animal's heart stopped beating. Now came the effort of butchering a huge animal, a task made easier with help, and two of the yak herder's neighbors had come to assist. Out here, *neighbor* is a relative term. Where I come from, *neighbor* would mean the person who lives in the house about 50 yards from mine, but on the steppe the nearest neighbor could be 30 miles away. These two made quite a journey to help their friend process this yak.

For most people in our society today, the butchering of an animal is at best confusing to watch, at worst disgusting and distressing. For me, it's fascinating. Why? Because it's an honest window into a society's diet and culture. Perspectives and values determine what parts of an animal are consumed and who consumes them. All of this, in turn, dictates how the animal is butchered. On the freezing steppe, I watched unorthodox butchering strategies unfold before me like none I'd ever seen before. At first, I was confused, but as they progressed, I began to understand that what these people valued from this animal was nothing like what we, in our Western culture, value.

With the exception of the spleen and gallbladder (which were fed to the dogs), nothing was wasted. With hands like surgeons, the herders worked together to remove the liver, heart, kidney, and lungs. The intestines would serve as casings for a sausage made of dried raw meat that would hang from the roof of the ger, enveloped in the dwelling's escaping smoke. The cleansed stomach would be filled with butter made from yak milk, where it would ferment for several months.

Once all of the blood and organs were removed, all surgical precision disappeared as the herders removed the meat. There were no prime cuts or subprime cuts or, for that matter, any recognizable individual cuts of meat, as there would be on our plates in the West. In fact, the meat was not removed from the bone at all. Everything — and I mean *everything* — that was left was chopped up together into fist-size chunks, each containing its own proportional share of meat, gristle, marrow, and fat. What was once a yak was now a pile of indiscernible pieces. Their butchering strategies and techniques clearly prioritized the most nutrient-dense part of the animal — the organs, blood, fat, and other offal — and were apathetic toward the meat. Making entirely different choices than a typical contemporary Western butcher for a contemporary Western consumer would, they achieved that zero-waste, nose-to-tail holy grail.

Why have I described this experience? Because it illustrates key points about the complicated and, at times, ethically charged question of how we consume meat in our contemporary Western culture. As with our relationship with plants, we need to rethink our relationship with animals. Most of us believe we are making a healthy choice when we go to the grocery store and purchase a pork tenderloin, some boneless, skinless breasts of chicken, or a thick New York strip steak. These are good choices, we are told, because they are lean cuts of meat, low in fat, high in protein. This isn't false information — these meats *are* relatively low in fat and high in protein. But it's not the whole story. In reality, we should be taking a cue from our ancestors and eating less meat and more animal.

By focusing only on meat — and especially lean meat — we have excluded nutritious, high-quality animal fats, organs, and other offal from our diets, and these are the most nutrient-dense, bioavailable foods on the planet for our human bodies. It's worth pausing here to address that word that makes many people squirm: *offal*. Likely derived from pre-16th-century Middle Dutch, the word traces its etymology to *af* (off) and *vallen* (fall) and literally means what falls out and off during the butchering process — that is, blood, organs, connective tissue, intestines, skin, and so on. Everything from sweetbreads (pancreas or thymus) to trotters (pig's feet), from tripe (stomach lining) to chitterlings (large intestine), can be considered offal. Something of a chameleon term, *offal* can mean different things in different foodways and cultures; in Western culture, it typically refers to the parts of the animal that are not considered food — pretty much everything that is not meat as we define it and that rarely, if ever, makes it to our tables. However, in this book, *offal* hews to its linguistic roots, meaning what it is: the organs, blood, fat, bones, skin, and other byproducts of the butchering process. The difference is that in this book those byproducts are considered valuable food.

By this definition, beef liver — something not entirely unheard of on Western plates — is offal, and it provides an illuminating nutritional comparison to the far more ubiquitous ground beef. A 100-gram serving of raw beef liver delivers 4.9 milligrams (mg) of iron, 313 mg of potassium, 9.8 mg of copper, 59 micrograms (mcg) of vitamin B_{12}, and a walloping 16,899 international units (IU) of vitamin A (in fact, eating too much liver can cause vitamin A toxicity). The same portion of ground beef contains 2 mg of iron, 175 mg of potassium, 0.1 mg of copper, 2 mcg of B_{12}, and zero vitamin A. They both deliver about the same amount of protein — 20.4 grams from the liver, 19.4 from the ground beef — while the liver is lower in calories (135 versus 192, respectively) and fat (3.6 grams versus 12.7). When we eat liver, our bodies easily absorb and use nearly all of the nutrition it contains. Meat, on the other hand, has fewer nutrients and requires processing (cooking) to make those nutrients completely bioavailable.

Yet despite all these undeniable attributes, liver is generally treated in our culinary world as something you smother with onions and serve (usually overcooked) for a blue-plate special at a diner. And it suffers from the common misconception that the liver stores toxins and therefore is toxic to eat. Rather, it breaks down and filters toxins. It, like other organ meats, has a marketing and perception problem, largely thanks to our current food system, which prioritizes meat while wasting the more useful and nutritious parts of an animal. In the United States, we eat approximately 55 percent of a pig by weight and 50 percent of a cow by weight. What ends up in the packages in the grocery store represents about half of the animal. The other half is either trashed or used for other products. And when we throw away half of an animal, we aren't only throwing away half of the nutrients it can provide; we're throwing away far more than that, because we are getting rid of the most nutrient-dense parts of the animal.

This emphasis on meat has warped our concept of what a truly healthy diet is in terms of animal protein. We are deathly afraid of fat. But high-quality animal fat literally helped fuel our most profound evolutionary advances as humans. Humans began eating meat by scavenging from dead animals whose viscera—the organs, blood, and fat—had already been stripped by predators. It took another 1.5 million years for us to develop the technology to hunt, and only then, after we were the first to a kill and were regularly eating the most nutritious parts, did our brains and bodies begin to grow exponentially. It wasn't the left-behind meat that did this; it was the rich, nutritious organs, fat, and other offal, parts that today are discarded, largely considered disgusting, and in some cases even made illegal. The great irony is that we have taken a gigantic step *backward* with our modern approach to meat. After our ancestors worked so hard to gain first access to an entire animal, today we are choosing the opposite strategy, eating the less nutritious parts of an animal and leaving the rest.

Why did this happen? There are a number of factors, but first and foremost we need to go back into the recent past — 1869 to be precise — when the Transcontinental Railroad was completed. This momentous accomplishment let us ship live animals across the country for eventual slaughter. But these animals took up a lot of space, they needed to be fed in transit, and they often lost weight or died during the stressful travel. To solve this problem, we came up with new refrigeration techniques that let us slaughter, butcher, and ship *meat* far more efficiently, economically, and safely from a few central locations — Chicago, Omaha, and Kansas City, for example. However, this new arrangement immediately took organ meats and other offal, which required more consistent, colder refrigeration than meat, off the table. It also resulted in the extinction of scores of local slaughterhouses and butchers across the country. The mountains of "waste" from the slaughterhouses — previously regarded as nutritionally dense foods — transformed into products like gelatin, grease, isinglass, and fertilizer. And thus the American diet shifted toward meat and away from offal, and we began what remains the practice today of eating only about half of the animal. This series of decisions, made solely for economic reasons, has resulted in our modern practice of eating only the flesh from select parts of an animal that has been slaughtered, butchered, packaged, and shipped by someone else. Not only does the average American play no role in any part of the process, most of us don't even know the butcher.

Interestingly, it's the middle class that seems to have the least physical and psychological access to offal. When raw offal is available, it's extremely inexpensive — in a typical American grocery store, a pound of liver costs about $2.50, versus about $10 a pound for a cut of meat like New York strip steak — and therefore it's more common in lower-income households. (Here's a nifty piece of offal trivia: The term *humble pie* derives from medieval times, when it meant a dish made of animal innards served in peasant households.) And in its finished form, offal is often presented at some of the world's finest (and priciest) restaurants as gorgeous and delicious pâtés and terrines. But it is not part of the diet of the average middle-class consumer. And while it's used in dishes throughout the world (from steak and kidney pie in England to gulai otak — brain curry — in Indonesia), only in more traditional cultures, such as the Sami, the Inuit, and the Mongolian yak herders I observed on the steppe, do organs, fat, and other offal continue to be the most consistently valued parts of the animal. The average American consumer, presented with a whole animal, wouldn't have a clue what to do with it. As with so many other aspects of our food culture, we have lost touch with those skills and processes that our great-grandparents and even in some cases our grandparents understood and used regularly.

So, how do we address our skewed relationship with animals as protein in our modern worlds and diets? As with much of our food, we need to shift our perceptions and our mindset. In the same way that we retooled our relationships with plants—by reestablishing a direct connection with our food, and then learning the technologies and processing methods to make it safe, nutrient-dense, and bioavailable—we can begin to return to the more sustainable, ethical, and healthy approach of eating more animal and less meat. As modern hunter-gatherers, we can forage wild plants, grow a garden, and source veggies from local markets and growers. When it comes to meat, we can apply the same practices: hunting, trapping, or fishing to obtain animals directly, or getting to know our local butcher or farmer and purchasing our meats there, including organs and other offal. While we use technologies like fermentation to make plants safe and bioavailable, we can learn the skills of nose-to-tail butchering and cooking to use *all* of the animal in ways that will not just satisfy but thrill our modern palates and nourish and satiate our bodies and, yes, souls. Before you say "No way, I can't butcher an animal" and close this book, I'm going to tell you that yes, you can, and you can do it right on your kitchen counter without much fuss. We'll get to that in a bit.

But first, a word about hunting. I realize that some people simply can't bring themselves to kill an animal. And even if they could, why bother with the effort? Our contemporary food system has made this decision easy for them. When we buy a plastic-wrapped piece of pork tenderloin at the grocery store and grill it over a bed of coals, it is a faceless, bloodless transaction. Most people consider this a perk of our modern food system. But for me, the opposite is true. I would argue that distancing ourselves from the process—by not knowing how that animal was raised, treated, fed, and killed—is fundamentally unethical and perpetuates a system that treats our food-producing animals atrociously and unsafely. Effectively removing ourselves from the things we don't want to be a part of doesn't mean they don't still happen. Rather, it means that they continue without us and, in the absence of our vigilant oversight, terrible situations and practices are enabled.

By accepting and supporting this system, we have nothing invested in the life or death of an animal that was killed to provide us with food. I'm not saying this to make anyone feel guilty or irresponsible; I am saying it to encourage us to think about the ethical imperative of putting a face on what we eat and to make a conscious choice to eliminate the distance between us and our food. Hunting is probably the most direct and accessible way to do this. Since I was a boy, learning the skills of hunting from my father in New Jersey, I have never liked the act of killing an animal, whether a squirrel, a goose, or a deer. But what I deeply, intensely appreciate is knowing that I have a direct connection to that animal, that I have killed it as quickly, painlessly, and respectfully as possible, that I will strive to waste none of it, and that I am certain it has been safely butchered and processed. As my father did for me, I have passed this knowledge along to my son, Billy, and it's immensely rewarding to see not only what a gifted hunter he has become, but also his skill and attention to the tasks that follow that make all the difference: field dressing, butchering, and cooking. When I witness his thoughtfulness toward an animal he has killed, it makes me proud to see how he understands why it is so important to make the most of every part of that animal, and how he approaches hunting—from start to finish— from that perspective. I realize that most people didn't grow up as I did with a knowledgeable and loving mentor who taught me all I needed to know to grow and evolve as a responsible, thoughtful hunter. But as the concept of direct sourcing of food becomes more mainstream, there are more and more opportunities to learn how to hunt and butcher wild game.

Still, if hunting simply isn't for you, the next best step is to find a local farmer or grower with whom you can develop a relationship. Learn how they raise their animals, what they feed them, how their animals live their lives. Many growers offer a share-purchase program similar to a CSA (community-supported agriculture) for produce; sign up, and you can be assured that you are getting meat that is ethically and locally grown and harvested. You will have taken a huge step toward putting a face to your food and drawing yourself closer to its source. If you don't have a farmer nearby, look for an artisan butcher, where access to organ meats such as liver, heart, and kidney is becoming easier.

Having grown up as I did, hunting with my dad, I thought I knew all there was to know about butchering and processing an animal to provide food for my family. But the truth is, only fairly recently did I learn about the nose-to-tail approach. For decades I had butchered animals the way I'd been taught—meaning, keeping the meat and discarding nearly every-thing else. But it was during a trip to Calabria, Italy, decades after my father had taught me to hunt, when I was able to truly learn how to put into practice what I had seen on the Mongolian steppe: a commitment to using all of an animal. It happened at the Italian Culinary Institute, where I spent a week under the tutelage of Chef John Nocita during his course in traditional Italian charcuterie and salumi and created a wide range of stun-ning, delicious foods, using traditional technologies, including ferment-ing, curing, and other innovative methods.

Notably, the course didn't begin in the classroom but rather at a farm, Casellone, where Calabrian black pigs are raised in a free-range, natural environment and fed a high-quality diet that includes the local olives. After we talked with the farmer and toured his farm, he invited us to choose two pigs that would be slaughtered for our class. This experience added a level of responsibility and significance to what we were doing. The pigs, dehaired, gutted, and split in half, arrived later that day. All of the organs and other offal were delivered separately in bags except for the intestines, which arrived in a five-gallon plastic bucket. From here, Chef John guided us in the different options we had that would inform how we would approach butchering each half. Once we began, we did not stop for the entire week. Between stories, lectures, demonstrations, and the ubiquitous "little snacks" John would provide, we prepped parts of the pig for fermen-tation, curing, and long-term storage. We cooked and ate on the spot parts such as the organs, skin, ears, and certain cuts of meat. We scraped and prepared the intestines that we would stuff for both fresh and fermented sausages. By the end of the course we had made a variety of whole-muscle cures, such as pancetta and prosciutto. We made lardo, or cured pig fat. We used the bones for bollito, or bone broth. We made fermented and cured meats, including salami and my personal favorite, 'nduja, a fermented and cured spicy spread made from all sorts of leftover bits that didn't meet the standards for other cured-meat products—a true zero-waste food that tastes absolutely delicious. We made a number of cooked dishes using everything—"choice" cuts of meat in pasta, pig skin in braciola, and odd bits and pieces in head cheese. We adhered to tradition but innovated when appropriate. By the end of the week, all that was left of the two pigs didn't even fill a medium bowl. Using traditional food-processing technologies, we transformed the animals into nutritious, delicious, gorgeous food that appealed to all of our senses and to which we all felt a close connection.

This experience was the quintessential nose-to-tail approach. Of course, not all of us can zoom off to Italy for a week to learn at the hands of a master. So, how to begin to achieve a nose-to-tail ethic in your own kitchen and in your relationship with animals in your diet? As with most things, small steps are the best way to start. You can attend butchering workshops or even find them online; I have developed a series of these, which are accessible to anyone with a computer. Or, you can just start with a whole chicken you buy at the store and butcher it yourself. Once you have mastered the chicken, go to the butcher and buy a whole pork shoulder, butcher it, and again use every part. Yes, you can do this on your kitchen counter! At this point in the butchering process, there is very little blood, since nearly all of it will have been removed at slaughter. Try roasting marrow for my Wild Greens, Roasted Bone Marrow, and Sourdough (page 38). Learn to cook kidneys. Make bone broth from the bones, pâtés and terrines from the organs, chicharrones from the skins, and rillettes from leftover cuts of meat, and keep leftover fats for daily cooking. As your skills grow, you can begin to cure meat. Make your own bacon—this is so much easier and more economical than you think—and even hot dogs and salami. Invite a neighbor or two to tackle butchering an entire half of a pig, making use of every single piece. Reconnect to your food, learn, empower yourself, have fun, and create change—all while feeding your body the most nourishing food on the planet.

TIPS AND RECIPES

COLOR-CODE YOUR CUTTING BOARDS

To avoid cross-contamination of flavors and pathogens, many professional kitchens use color-coded cutting boards—red for raw meat, green for vegetables, brown for cooked meat, yellow for poultry, white for bread, and blue for fish and seafood. This is a great idea for your home kitchen, too. In my home kitchen, we have separate color-coded cutting boards for raw meat, garlic and onions, all other vegetables, and sourdough bread.

BUTCHER AT HOME

Directly accessing whole or large parts of animals is not as difficult as you may think. If you have a local butcher, great, but even if you don't, you can find whole chickens at farmer's markets, most grocery stores, and even big-box, bulk-food, chain stores like Costco or BJ's. Follow the instructions below and check out eatlikeahuman.com for tutorials on home butchery.

SAVE THE FAT

Any time you cook an animal—a chicken, steak, bacon—there is leftover fat. Most of us just scrape it into the garbage can, but you should save it. This nutrient-dense, satiating, and delicious animal fat can be used in place of oil or butter for cooking. It is, in fact, much safer to use in high-heat cooking than nut and seed oils, which break down at high temperatures and release harmful free radicals. This is fat that has been rendered during the cooking process, so it can safely stay at room temperature, which makes it easy to use every day. I keep several jars on the side of my stove — one with lard, one with bacon grease, and one with schmaltz (poultry fat).

FREEZE UNTIL YOU HAVE ENOUGH

It makes sense to cook in bulk. Most animal parts — fat, bones, and organs — freeze very well. I always keep several resealable bags in the freezer at all times:

- Chicken livers: Each time I butcher a chicken, I add the liver to the bag. I defrost when I have accumulated enough to make pâté.
- Bones and carcasses: When I do anything with animals (butchering, roasting, boiling, grilling), I add the bones to the bones bag. When I have enough, I make a big batch of bone broth. You can keep separate bags for the bones of different animals or put them all together; this is a personal preference depending on the type of bone broth you want to make.
- Raw fat: Fat that has not yet been cooked can be set aside for later rendering. The freezer is an ideal place to store this raw fat. I defrost and use it once I have enough to render. As with bones, you can store fat from different animals either in different bags or in the same bag, depending on whether you plan to render it separately or together.

KEEP THE VEGGIES FOR BONE BROTH

When I trim vegetables — cut the ends off carrots, celery, and onions; peel carrots; and take the skin off onions — I put all those scraps in a resealable bag that I keep in the freezer. Each time I prep veggies I add to this bag, and when I'm ready to make bone broth, I use those scraps instead of wasting whole vegetables. However, trimmings from some vegetables, such as rutabagas, bell peppers, and members of the Brassica family (for example, broccoli, cauliflower, and cabbage), should be avoided as they can produce strong, off flavors. Never use potato peels, as they contain toxins that can leach into the water. Experiment and see what works best for you.

HEALTHY DEEP FRYING? YES!

Deep-frying food creates incredible flavors, aromas, and textures. But can it be healthy? Absolutely. The following steps explain how to make the most of deep frying in your kitchen:

1. Use only saturated fats such as lard and tallow for deep frying. Avoid using vegetable or nut and seed oils.
2. Some deep fryers are specially designed for frying in animal fat, but any will work as long as you melt the fat before filling.
3. If you do not have a deep fryer, use a heavy-duty pot, fill no more than halfway with fat, and use a thermometer clipped to the side to keep track of the temperature.
4. Most foods, like fried chicken, can be deep-fried successfully at 350°F. However, a few foods benefit from different temperatures and techniques. Use the following temperature guidelines for optimal results:

    Chips (potato and tortilla): Fry at 300°F. The lower temperature allows the chips to dehydrate before browning and results in a crispier chip. (See Lacto-Chips, page 57, and Tortilla Chips, page 162.)

    French fries: The best French fries are fried twice; the first fry cooks them and the second browns and crisps them. Fry at 325°F for 5 minutes. Drain and cool completely, then fry at 375°F for 2 to 3 minutes, until brown. (See Lacto-Fries, page 58.)

    Pork rinds: Fry at 375°F until puffy. Since they have already been dehydrated, they can be cooked at a higher temperature. (See Pork Rinds, page 93.)

WHY CHICKEN? AN ACCESSIBLE
NOSE-TO-TAIL APPROACH

A true nose-to-tail approach does not require you to start hunting, nor does it mean you have to drag half a pig into your home and butcher it on your countertop (although, take it from me, that is a rewarding experience!). Rather, with a simple mindset shift and a few basic skills, you can approach something as simple as a whole chicken in a more ethical, sustainable, nourishing, and economical way. Make sure to purchase the highest-quality chicken possible. This ensures that you are not only feeding your family nourishing food, but you are also supporting the farmers, abattoirs, and butchers who are doing excellent work. Since you will be using every part of the chicken, the cost gets spread out over more than just one meal and makes that high-quality chicken more affordable.

Here are the steps to butchering a chicken:

1. Set up your workstation: You should have a cutting board sitting on top of a damp paper towel to keep it from moving, a sharp knife (preferably a boning knife), a small bowl for the organs, a large bowl for bone broth ingredients, and a large platter for meat (see Figure 1).

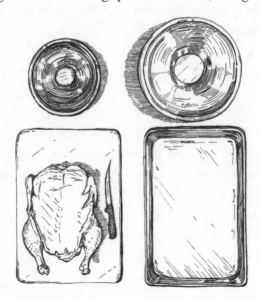

Figure 1

2. Remove the innards, if present: Stick your hand inside the cavity and remove the liver, heart, gizzard, and neck (see Figure 2). Put the organs you are reserving to cook separately (such as the liver and heart) in the small bowl. Put everything else in the large bowl for bone broth.

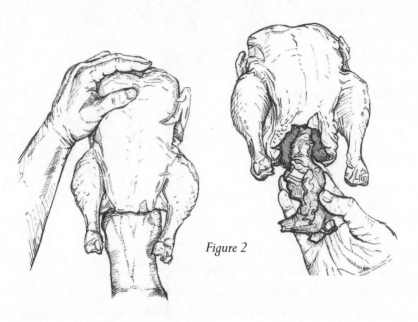

Figure 2

3. Remove the legs: Place your knife on the inside of one leg with the blade parallel to the body. Slice through the skin and carefully separate the leg from the body, keeping the knife close to the body until you get to the ball joint (see Figure 3a). Using your free hand, pull the leg away from the body until the ball snaps

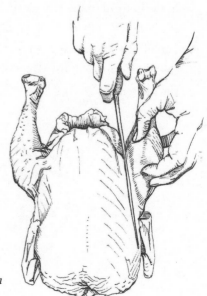

Figure 3a

free from the joint.
Continue to follow
the body with the
knife to separate the
remaining portion
of the leg (see
Figure 3b). Repeat
with the other leg.
Put the legs on the
platter.

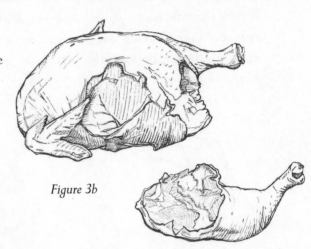

Figure 3b

4. Remove the wings: Turn the chicken over so that the back is
    facing up. Beginning on the underside of the joint
    where the wing meets the body, slice through the
    skin and under the joint, following the contour
    of the body until the wing is separated from
    the body (see Figure 4). Take care not to
    cut into the breast meat. Repeat with
    the other wing. Put the wings on
    the platter.

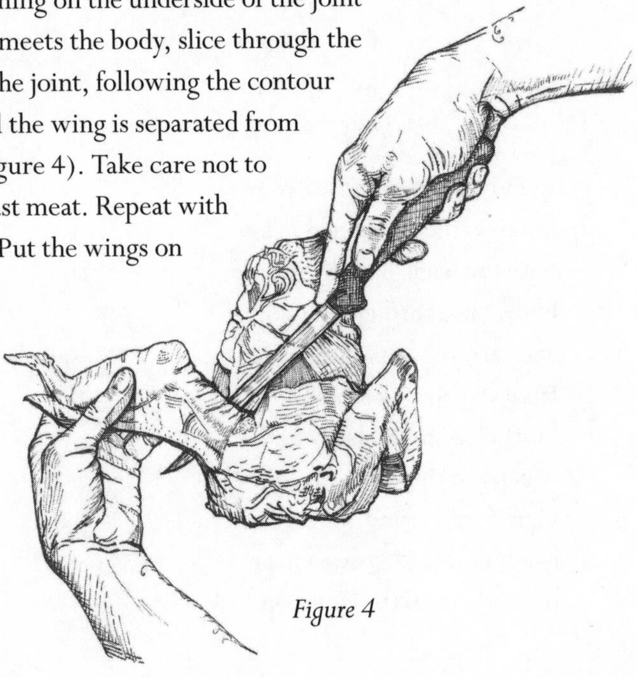

Figure 4

5. Disarticulate the legs: Hold the end of one drumstick in one hand and cut to the inside of the joint between the drumstick and the thigh with your knife. Flex the joint to separate the bones; ensure that the knife is in the correct position and continue the cut with the knife to separate the drumstick from the thigh (see Figure 5a). Repeat with the other leg. Return the drumsticks and thighs to the platter. Next, hold a wing by one end and begin the cut between the drumette and wingette on the inside of the joint. Flex the joint to separate the bones; ensure that the knife is in the correct position and continue the cut with the knife (see Figure 5b). Do the same thing to separate the wingette and the wing tip. Repeat with the other wing. Put the wing tips in the large bowl for bone broth and return the other wing pieces to the platter.

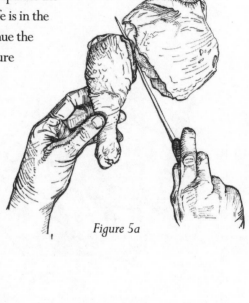

Figure 5a

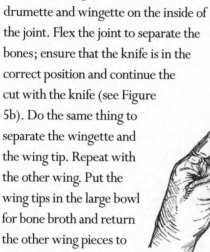

Figure 5b

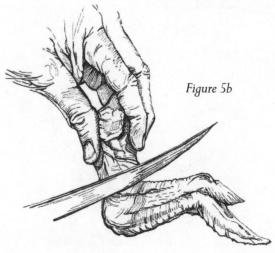

6. Remove the wishbone: Place the chicken with the breast facing up and the neck area toward you. Locate the wishbone with your finger; it will be at the front of the breast, just under a thin layer of meat. With your knife held vertically, cut along the back side of the wishbone to free it from both breasts (see Figure 6a). This should be a shallow cut that extends only to the bottom of the wishbone. Using your fingers, find the center of the wishbone and pull it toward you (see Figure 6b). Use the knife to free the bone from each end and anywhere it is still attached. Put the wishbone in the large bowl.

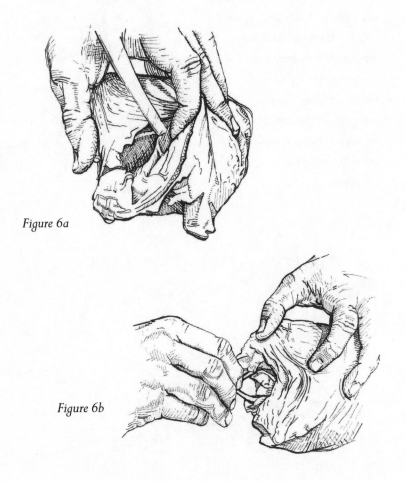

Figure 6a

Figure 6b

7. Remove the breasts and separate the tenders from the breast meat:
   With the legs, wings, and wishbone removed, you have full access
   to the breast. Turn the chicken, still breast side up, so that the
   neck area is facing away from you. Locate the breastbone; it is a
   bony ridge running lengthwise between the breasts. Make a cut
   with your knife straight down on either side of the bone. Extend
   this cut down the breastbone until your knife comes in contact
   with the ribs (see Figure 7a). Turn your knife 90 degrees and

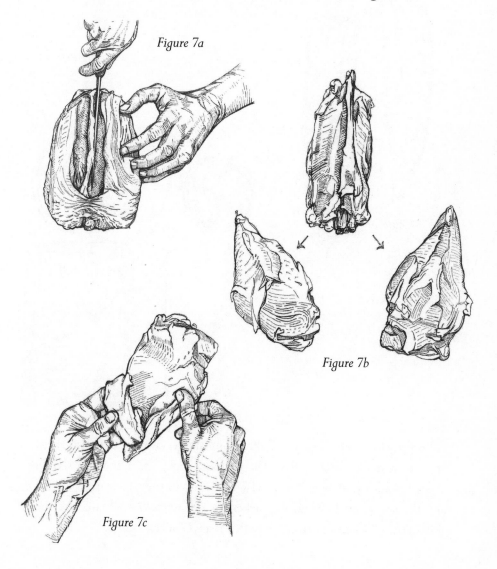

Figure 7a

Figure 7b

Figure 7c

follow the ribs to remove each breast. Each breast will have a flap of meat on the underside (see Figure 7b). These are the tenders and, if you like, you can remove them by pulling them away from the breast (see Figure 7c). Put the breast and tenders (see Figure 7d) on the platter and the carcass in the large bowl (see Figure 7e).

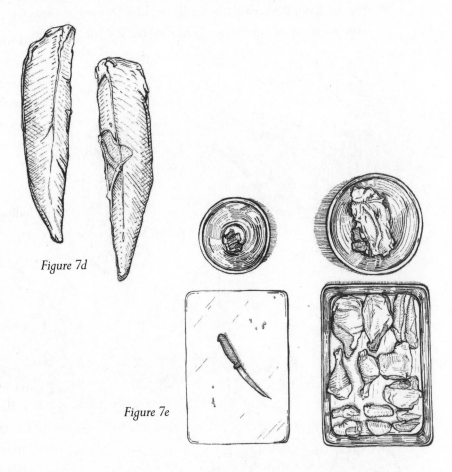

Figure 7d

Figure 7e

Following are some recipes to make the most of every part of the chicken, and not just the meaty parts. The carcass, neck, and wing tips should always go into your bone broth. Use the livers in the Chicken Liver Pâté and the hearts in the Grilled Chicken Hearts with Wild Pesto. Use the skin in the Chicken Caesar Salad with Crispy Chicken Skins.

TRASH BONE BROTH

Makes about 1 gallon

A hot mug of bone broth just might be one of the most nourishing and comforting foods on the planet. This is a simple and versatile approach to making bone broth from all of your butchering scraps. If in doubt, throw it in. Although the recipe calls for chicken bones, it also works great with turkey, goose, duck, pig, cow, and even deer. You can use raw bones as well as the leftover bones from cooking. However, bones from mammals make particularly good bone broth when they have been roasted, so I usually roast raw bones in a 400°F oven, turning occasionally until they are browned, before throwing them in the pot.

> 1 chicken carcass, either raw or left over from roasting, including
> bones, cartilage, connective tissue, neck, backbone, heart,
> and feet (if you have them)
> 2 tablespoons apple cider vinegar
> 2 to 5 whole black peppercorns
> 1 bay leaf
> Vegetable scraps (optional)

If you have chicken feet, wash them well, then use a meat cleaver or kitchen shears to cut them into several pieces, as they release their collagen most efficiently this way. Put all the chicken parts in a large pot. Cover everything with cold water and add the apple cider vinegar. Allow to sit for 30 to 60 minutes. The vinegar helps draw valuable minerals from the bones into the bone broth. If you skip this step, it is not the end of the world, but it's worth doing if you have the time.

Add the peppercorns and bay leaf. Bring to a boil over medium-high heat, skim any foam that rises to the surface, then cover and reduce to a simmer over low heat. You can simmer for as little as 1 hour or up to 12 hours for a more flavorful and nutritious broth. If you are adding vegetable scraps, do so during the last hour of cooking. Cooking vegetables for too long will result in a bitter bone broth.

When you have finished simmering, strain the bone broth through a fine-mesh strainer and discard the solids. Let the broth cool, then transfer to a jar, cover, and store in the refrigerator for up to 1 week or in the freezer for up to 6 months.

CHICKEN LIVER PÂTÉ

Pâté is sort of a "gateway organ meat" and is perhaps the most accessible way to transform the initially off-putting visuals, textures, and strong odors of offal into something that looks and tastes delicious. I never advocate hiding or sneaking foods into dishes as a way to mask what someone is actually eating, as doing so undermines the goal of connecting people with their food. Rather, it's all about context: A well-plated, fine-textured pâté presented with homemade sourdough bread should elicit a completely different response from an "in-your-face" whole organ sitting on a plate, no matter how expertly prepared. This easy-to-prepare pâté is a great way to use up those chicken livers you have been storing in your freezer.

1 cup (2 sticks) butter, divided
2 garlic cloves, chopped
1 tablespoon fresh thyme leaves, plus an optional sprig for garnish
8 ounces chicken livers, washed and trimmed
2 tablespoons brandy
Sea salt and freshly ground black pepper
Bay leaf (optional)

Cut ½ cup (1 stick) of the butter into ½-inch cubes. Put the cubes of butter in the fridge to keep cold.

Melt the remaining ½ cup (1 stick) butter in a small saucepan over low heat. Add the garlic and thyme leaves and cook over low heat for 5 minutes to infuse the butter with the flavor and aroma of the garlic and thyme, then turn off the heat. Place a fine-mesh strainer over a small bowl. Skim the butter of any foam that may have risen to the top, and put this foam in a blender. Slowly pour the clarified butter through the strainer, leaving the white milky sediment behind in the saucepan. Add that sediment to the blender, along with the garlic and thyme from the strainer.

Ladle a tablespoon of the clarified butter into a frying pan and heat over medium heat. When the pan is hot, add the livers and cook for a couple of minutes on each side, until just barely pink inside (poke one with a knife to check). Add the livers to the blender. Turn the heat to medium-high and deglaze the pan with the brandy, using a wooden spoon to dislodge any bits sticking to the pan. Scrape into the blender.

Turn on the blender and process until smooth. Allow to cool until warm but no longer hot. Add the cubed butter from the refrigerator and process again until smooth. Season with salt and pepper to taste. Push the pâté through a fine-mesh strainer with a spatula to ensure a smooth consistency. Distribute into ramekins or small jars. Make sure there are no air pockets in the pâté and the surface is as flat and even as possible. Use a damp paper towel to wipe any residual pâté from the sides of the ramekins.

If you want to kick the presentation up a notch, place a sprig of thyme or a bay leaf on top of the pâté. Pour a thin layer of clarified butter on top. Carefully transfer to the fridge and cool until the butter is hardened. Bring to room temperature and serve, or cover with plastic wrap and store in the fridge for up to 1 week or in the freezer for several months. Any leftover clarified butter can be stored in a covered container in the fridge for up to 1 month.

GRILLED CHICKEN HEARTS WITH WILD PESTO

Serves 4

Animal hearts are nutritional powerhouses. Since they are essentially muscles, their flavor and texture are more familiar to us than the flavors and textures of other organ meats, so they are a great place to start as you explore organ meats. Plus, they are delicious. Keep a resealable bag in your freezer for storing hearts each time you butcher a chicken. When you have enough saved up, use this simple recipe to serve them to your family.

> 8 ounces chicken hearts
> Sea salt
> ¼ cup Wild Pesto (page 41) or any pesto

Preheat the grill to medium-high.

Thread the chicken hearts onto skewers and salt liberally. Grill on both sides until cooked through, about 10 minutes total. Brush with the pesto while still warm and serve.

GRANNY'S CHICKEN

SERVES 4

I grew up in Shrewsbury, New Jersey, only a few miles from the beach. On Sundays, my maternal grandmother would pack a picnic dinner and the entire family would head to Sandy Hook Beach late in the afternoon, well after the crowds had left. With the beach practically to ourselves, we would surf, fish, fly kites, and enjoy Granny's chicken, the highlight of the meal. Perhaps it is because of the memories, but to this day I like this chicken better cold. Here is a version of her recipe, altered slightly to make it even more nourishing.

> 2 cups sourdough breadcrumbs
> ½ cup grated Parmesan cheese
> 1 teaspoon sea salt
> ½ teaspoon garlic powder
> 1 cup Fermented Butter (see page 189), melted
> 4 chicken drumsticks
> 4 chicken thighs

Preheat the oven to 350°F. Lightly grease a rimmed baking sheet.

Thoroughly combine the breadcrumbs, cheese, salt, and garlic powder in a wide, shallow dish. Put the melted butter in another dish. Dip the chicken pieces first in the melted butter, then roll them in the breadcrumb mixture. Place skin side up on the prepared baking sheet and bake for 1 hour, or until the internal temperature reads 165°F. Serve warm, or let cool, then wrap tightly and refrigerate to serve chilled the next day.

FRIED CHICKEN WINGS

Believe it or not, chicken wings can be nourishing, ethically responsible, and delicious. Just think about it: The drumettes and wingettes are byproducts of chicken butchering, so using them helps support a nose-to-tail, zero-waste approach. And, eating them provides our bodies with nourishment not just from the meat but also from the skin and connective tissue. Despite their healthy potential, though, almost all the chicken wings you buy at a restaurant are harmful because they're made of mass-produced chicken fried in unhealthy industrial nut and seed oils. To make matters worse, when we eat them, we dip the wings in blue cheese and ranch dressings made from the same nut and seed oils. Making these wings entirely from scratch ensures that you have control over the process and can use high-quality chicken, fry in lard or tallow, and make your blue cheese dressing with avocado oil. Add home-fermented carrot sticks to complete this nourishing twist on an otherwise unhealthy junk food.

> 6 whole chicken wings (or 12 drumette/wingette pieces)
> 2 quarts animal fat (such as lard or tallow)
> ⅓ cup hot sauce
> ⅓ cup butter, melted
> Fermented Carrot Sticks (page 52), for serving
> Bola's Blue Cheese Dressing (page 87), for serving

Preheat the oven to 350°F.

Separate the drumettes, wingettes, and tips. Reserve the tips for making Trash Bone Broth, page 79. Arrange the drumettes and wingettes on a rimmed baking sheet and bake for 45 minutes, turning halfway through. Transfer the wings to a cooling rack and cool thoroughly. These steps are essential to creating the crispiest and most delicious wings possible. Once the wings are cool, they can be fried and eaten or frozen for long-term storage. If you are freezing them, arrange them on a tray so that they're not touching and freeze thoroughly before packing them together in bulk. They can be deep-fried directly from the freezer, and freezing them separately lets you remove only what you need.

When you are ready for the final cooking, heat the animal fat to 375°F in a deep fryer or large, heavy pot. Add the wings to the hot fat and fry until the skin reaches the desired crispiness and color, 3 to 5 minutes. Since they are already cooked, all you need to do is crisp the outside and warm the middle. Drain on a cooling rack, a crumpled brown paper bag, or paper towels. Mix together the hot sauce and melted butter in a large container with a lid. While the wings are still warm, place them in the container with the sauce, cover, and shake to coat the wings. Serve with carrot sticks and blue cheese dressing on the side.

BOLA'S BLUE CHEESE DRESSING

MAKES ABOUT 2 CUPS

Christina and I met while working at the Alchemist and Barrister, a restaurant in Princeton, New Jersey. In fact, we started our first shifts on the same night—I was the new bartender and she was the new waitress. Bola, one of the chefs, made an amazing blue cheese dressing. To this day it is hands down the best blue cheese dressing I have ever tasted. The secret is to take half the blue cheese and blend it into the dressing to fully incorporate the flavor. This version uses homemade omega-3–rich mayonnaise (Omega-naise, page 88) and fermented cream to maximize the flavor and nutrition.

> 1 cup Omega-naise (recipe follows) or highest-quality store-bought mayonnaise
> ½ cup crumbled blue cheese, divided
> ½ cup Fermented Cream (page 187) or sour cream
> 1 tablespoon freshly squeezed lemon juice
> 1 teaspoon Worcestershire sauce
> ½ teaspoon sea salt
> Freshly ground black pepper

Beat together the mayonnaise, half of the blue cheese, the fermented cream, lemon juice, Worcestershire sauce, and salt with a hand mixer or whisk until smooth. Fold in the remaining blue cheese with a silicone spatula. Season with pepper to taste. Store in a sealed jar in the refrigerator for up to 1 week.

Omega-naise

MAKES ABOUT 3 CUPS

My younger daughter, Alyssa, loves mayonnaise on everything. If it is my homemade mayonnaise, I let her eat as much as she wants. Almost all commercial mayonnaise is made with industrial nut and seed oils and has no place in a healthy diet. However, substituting pure avocado oil transforms a food that can cause harm into a food that can nourish. Avocado oil is the fat of choice for mayonnaise in our house because it has a relatively low amount of omega-6 (a fatty acid that is way too prevalent in our modern diets) and an abundant amount of omega-9 (oleic acid), is minimally processed, and possesses a neutral flavor perfectly suited for mayonnaise. Feel free to replace up to half of the avocado oil with extra virgin olive oil or even room-temperature melted lard or unsalted butter. Just make sure to establish the emulsion with the avocado or olive oil first. You can make this recipe with a hand mixer, food processor, countertop blender, or stick blender. Unless I am making huge quantities, I still like to do it by hand with a whisk. The feel of a whisk in your hand, as you convert egg yolks and oil into something special, is especially satisfying.

> 3 large egg yolks
> 2 garlic cloves, minced (optional)
> 1 teaspoon Fermented Mustard (page 103) or Dijon mustard
> Sea salt
> 2 cups avocado oil
> 2 teaspoons white wine vinegar, or more if needed
> Juice of 1 lemon

Set a medium bowl on top of a kitchen towel or moistened paper towel on the counter. This will help keep the bowl from moving as you whisk. Put the egg yolks, garlic (if using), mustard, and a pinch of salt in the bowl and whisk together. Gradually add about half the oil, very slowly at first, drop by drop, while whisking continuously. Once the emulsion is established, increase the flow of oil into a thin stream. After you have added about half the oil, whisk in the vinegar; this will loosen the mixture slightly, making it easier to incorporate the remainder of the oil. Continue to gradually add the remaining oil, whisking continuously. Season with another pinch of salt, the lemon juice, and a little more vinegar, if needed. Store in a sealed jar in the fridge for up to 1 week.

CHICKEN CAESAR SALAD WITH CRISPY CHICKEN SKINS

SERVES 4

Every family milestone, from anniversaries to tenure, was celebrated at our favorite local restaurant, Brooks Tavern. All of the food there was terrific, but the highlight was the Caesar salad topped with a combination of bread-crumbs and Parmesan cheese and placed under the broiler just long enough to toast the top and barely wilt the edges of the romaine. Unfortunately, the restaurant is no longer open, but the head chef/owner, Kevin McKin-ney, shared his recipe with me, and with his permission, I am sharing a slightly modified version here. Make the mayonnaise for the dressing from scratch to elevate this delicious meal to its most nourishing form possible.

2 tablespoons extra virgin olive oil, plus more for greasing

2 boneless, skin-on chicken breasts

Sea salt and freshly ground black pepper

2 heads romaine lettuce

½ cup Brooks' Caesar Dressing (recipe follows)

¼ cup grated Parmesan cheese

½ cup sourdough breadcrumbs

Preheat the oven to 375°F. Line a rimmed baking sheet with parch-ment paper and coat lightly with olive oil.

Pull the skin off each chicken breast in one piece, remove any excess fat and meat from the skin, and return the chicken to the fridge. Cut each piece of skin in half to create a total of four pieces. Arrange the chicken skins on the prepared baking sheet, then cover with another piece of parchment paper that has been lightly coated with olive oil. Top with another baking sheet to weigh it down.

Bake for 40 to 50 minutes, until crisp. Drain the skin on paper towels and season to taste with salt and pepper while still warm. Set aside.

Preheat the grill to medium-high.

Season the chicken breasts with salt and pepper and grill, turning once, until they reach an internal temperature of 165°F, about 10 minutes. Cover loosely with aluminum foil or an upside-down bowl to rest.

Turn the oven broiler to high with a rack in the top position.

Wash and thoroughly dry the romaine lettuce. Tear into bite-size pieces and place in a bowl. Add dressing and toss to coat, then arrange on a heatproof platter. Combine the grated Parmesan cheese, sourdough breadcrumbs, and olive oil in a medium bowl and stir. Evenly top the lettuce with the mixture.

Place the platter under the broiler to toast the cheese and breadcrumb mixture. This will take only a few minutes, so watch carefully; under the intense direct heat of the broiler the transition from brown to burnt takes only a few seconds. Divide the salad onto four plates. Slice the chicken breasts and arrange on top of the salads. Garnish with the crispy chicken skin.

Brooks' Caesar Dressing

MAKES ABOUT 4 CUPS

½ cup extra virgin olive oil

¼ cup plus 2 tablespoons freshly squeezed lemon juice

2 tablespoons Fermented Mustard (page 103) or Dijon mustard

1 tablespoon Worcestershire sauce

3 garlic cloves, peeled

5 anchovy fillets

1 tablespoon freshly ground black pepper

2½ cups Omega-naise (page 88) or highest-quality store-bought
    mayonnaise

Combine the olive oil, lemon juice, mustard, Worcestershire, garlic, anchovies, and pepper in a blender and blend until smooth. Use a silicone spatula to scrape the contents of the blender into a large bowl. Add the mayonnaise and whisk to combine. Store in a sealed jar in the refrigerator for up to 2 weeks.

PORK RINDS

SERVES 4

Sure, pork rinds are a fantastic go-to snack for anyone restricting their carbohydrate intake, but did you know they are also high in protein and collagen? And, by preparing them by frying in lard or tallow, you are also introducing high-quality animal fat. They are easy to make yourself and far superior in nutrition and flavor to anything you can buy. In addition to salt, you can add all sorts of spices, from garlic powder to Old Bay seasoning. Ask your local butcher for pork skin or order it online.

1 pound pork skin
2 quarts animal fat (such as lard or tallow)
Sea salt

Bring a medium pot of water to a boil over medium-high heat. Trim the pork skin of any fat and connective tissue that are easily removed. Don't spend too much time trying to get every last bit; it will be removed more easily after it is boiled. Cut the skin into 1½-inch-wide strips. Add the strips to the boiling water, cover, and reduce the heat to maintain a low boil. Boil for 1 hour.

Carefully remove the skin from the water with tongs and place on a cutting board to cool slightly. Once the skins are cool enough to handle, use a plastic scraper to scrape away any remaining fat.

Dehydrate the skins in your oven at its lowest setting (for most of us that is 170°F) until they are completely dry and brittle, about 8 hours. At this point the dehydrated skins can be fried immediately or stored in an airtight container at room temperature for several months and fried later.

When you are ready to fry, pour the animal fat into a deep fryer or large, heavy pot and heat to 375°F. While the fat is heating, break the dehydrated skin into 1½-inch squares. Deep-fry the pork rinds until they expand, float, and just barely begin to brown. Drain on a cooling rack, a crumpled brown paper bag, or paper towels. Season with salt while still warm. Once cooled, they can be eaten right away or stored in an airtight container at room temperature for up to 1 week.

BACK FAT CRACKLINS

Okay...I like to snack on pork rinds, but I absolutely *love* everything about back fat cracklins. They deliver the same nutrition as pork rinds along with a healthy serving of nourishing fat. The flavor is fantastic, and perhaps the best part is the texture. When cooked properly, the skin is crunchy while the fat is creamy. The trick, however, is getting the skin to crisp while not burning the fat. You achieve this by starting with a cold pan and slowly increasing the heat to allow the skins to completely dehydrate and tenderize before they are overcooked.

> 1 pound skin-on pork back fat with a fat layer at least ¼ inch thick
> Sea salt

With a sharp knife, trim the fat to an even ¼-inch thickness (reserve the fat you cut off for rendering). Cut the pork into strips measuring approximately 1 inch by ¼ inch. Place the pieces, fat side down, in a cold sauté pan, turn the heat to low, and cook slowly, stirring occasionally to dehydrate and tenderize and crisp the skin. The cracklins are done when the skin begins to swell and pop and they are golden brown, 30 minutes to 1 hour.

Drain and season with salt while still warm. Store in an airtight container at room temperature for up to 1 week.

RENDERING LARD AND TALLOW

There are many different ways to obtain high-quality fat from animals—from cooking bacon and saving the grease to skimming the fat that rises to the top of a well-made bone broth. But there is something special and versatile about rendering pure fat from animals to store and use in all sorts of recipes.

> 5 pounds pork and/or beef fat
> 1 cup water

Preheat the oven to 250°F.

Remove any skin, meat, and connective tissue from the fat. Dice the fat into 1-inch pieces; this increases the surface area to allow for even and consistent heating. Put the fat in a Dutch oven or other ovenproof pot and add the water. (Adding water prevents burning until some fat has rendered; it will evaporate during the process.) Place the pot, uncovered, in the oven and cook, stirring occasionally, until the fat has rendered. Depending on the amount of fat and the size you cut the fat into, this could take several hours. Once the fat is rendered, strain and pour it into individual mason jars to cool. Once cool, cover tightly and store away from light at room temperature for up to 1 month, in the refrigerator for up to 3 months, or in the freezer for up to 1 year. Reserve the cracklins in a covered container in the fridge for up to 3 months. Reheat and brown them in a skillet, and use for topping salads, appetizers, and anywhere a rich crunch is needed.

MODERN STONE AGE KITCHEN BACON

MAKES ABOUT 8 POUNDS

Bacon gets a bad rap, and it should, but not for the reason you may think. The fat in bacon is actually a nutritional powerhouse and something we should celebrate. The problem is that most commercially available bacon is complete junk. It is made from the bellies of mass-produced pigs raised in inhumane conditions, is chock-full of nitrates, nitrites, and other preservatives, and is often injected with water to increase the weight and jack up the price. Unfortunately, higher-quality bacon is so expensive it is out of reach for most consumers. The good news is that bacon is easy and safe to make at home. Plus, by making it from scratch, you control the entire process, from where the meat comes from to what goes into it. My family absolutely loves bacon. After all, what's not to love? They eat as much as they want, as long as it is homemade.

You will need a scale, a vacuum sealer, and a smoker to make this bacon. If you don't own these, ask to borrow them from a neighbor. Believe me, making this bacon is worth the effort; just make sure to give your neighbor a pack of bacon when you return the equipment! Of course, if you do not have access to a smoker, then go ahead and cook the belly in your oven using the instructions below for the smoker. Your bacon won't be smoked but will still be nourishing and delicious.

> 114 grams sea salt
> 114 grams unrefined sugar (such as Sucanat or muscovado)
> 10 pounds skin-on pork belly (aka fresh side)
> Whiskey, white wine, or other alcohol for rinsing

Mix the salt and sugar in a small bowl and rub all over the belly, making sure to concentrate on the surfaces not covered by skin. Cut the belly into portions to fit inside vacuum bags, and vacuum-seal them to remove air. Refrigerate for 10 days to cure.

At the end of the curing phase, remove the belly pieces from the bags, rinse with alcohol to remove excess salt and sugar, and hang in a cool, breezy location or set in the fridge, uncovered, for a few hours so the surface dries and forms a skin known as a pellicle. This pellicle helps the smoke adhere to the bacon. Hot-smoke the belly pieces at 170°F until they reach an internal temperature of 145°F. This will take several hours, depending on the thickness of the belly and the type of smoker.

Remove the belly pieces from the smoker, allow to cool completely, and wrap tightly with plastic wrap. Refrigerate for 24 hours for the flavors to mellow. Slice them with a meat slicer or a very sharp knife. The bacon can be cooked immediately or wrapped tightly and stored in the fridge for up to 1 week or in the freezer for several months.

Notes:

This recipe is adaptable to any size belly. The ratio is 2.5% salt and 2.5% sugar calculated against the weight of the belly. To calculate the amount of salt and sugar, simply weigh the belly in grams and multiply by 0.25.

You don't need to use sugar. If you omit the sugar, use 3% salt instead of 2.5%.

Get creative! You can add all sorts of herbs and spices to the salt and sugar. Black peppercorns, dried rosemary, and red pepper flakes are excellent choices.

THE ULTIMATE NOSE-TO-TAIL BURGER

MAKES 4 BURGERS

Burgers are an American classic. When made from healthy beef raised on grass, they are an excellent source of protein and fat. Some people also use them as a more palatable way to include organ meats in their diets. While I am not a fan of disguising food, the ability to grind different parts and put them back together provides an opportunity to create a powerhouse of nutrients that also represents an ancestral nose-to-tail approach to animals. Grinding and cooking also make the meat's nutrients more bioavailable. In developing this recipe, I calculated the breakdown of the different parts of beef cattle and created a burger with a ratio of meat (70 percent), fat (17 percent), and organs (13 percent) that is reflective of the entire animal.

Meat grinder attachments for stand mixers are relatively affordable, and hand-crank meat grinders are cheap and easy to find at secondhand stores. Many small butchers will custom grind for their customers. Alternatively, you can completely skip the grinding step by finely mincing the raw organs and adding them along with the herbs and spices in the recipe below to 1 pound of already ground grass-fed beef (80 percent lean, 20 percent fat).

> 1 pound boneless chuck or other beef (80:20 lean-to-fat ratio)
> 2½ ounces organs (any combination of heart, liver, spleen, and/or kidneys)
> 1 garlic clove, minced
> 1 teaspoon smoked paprika
> ¼ teaspoon onion powder
> ¼ teaspoon sea salt
> ½ teaspoon freshly ground black pepper
> 1 tablespoon Worcestershire sauce

For serving (optional)

>4 Airfield Sourdough Bread buns (page 135), toasted if desired
>
>Modern Stone Age Kitchen Bacon (page 97), cooked
>
>Lettuce leaves
>
>Tomato and/or onion slices
>
>Fermented Ketchup (page 101)
>
>Fermented Mustard (page 103)

Cut the meat, fat, and organs into 1-inch cubes, spread them out on a tray, and freeze for 30 minutes. This will help ensure the fat does not smear during the grinding. Remove from the freezer and grind through an electric grinder or hand grinder into a medium bowl, using the plate attachment with the largest holes. Add the remaining ingredients, mix well by hand, and place the bowl in the freezer so that the meat remains cold while you switch over to the medium-grind plate.

When the grinder is ready, remove the ground meat from the freezer and grind one more time. Form into four equal patties. The burgers are ready to grill, or you can store them, tightly wrapped, in the refrigerator for up to 3 days or in the freezer for up to 3 months.

When ready to grill, preheat the grill to medium-high.

Grill the burgers, turning once, until cooked to your preference, about 10 minutes. Serve on buns with all your favorite fixings.

Note:

If you have access to a variety of organs, here is the breakdown of the ideal nose-to-tail burger: 13 ounces lean beef, 2 ounces fat, 1 ounce marrow, 1 ounce liver, ¾ ounce heart, ½ ounce kidney, ¼ ounce spleen.

FERMENTED KETCHUP

MAKES ABOUT 2 CUPS

My first taste of archaeology happened when I was a kid and my father unearthed a bunch of very cool old bottles while digging up our front yard to fix a water pipe leak. We later discovered that these tiny bottles were ketchup bottles from E. C. Hazard and Company, which once existed on the same spot. At its peak at the turn of the 20th century, Hazard generated annual revenues between $7 and $9 million and even helped introduce Tabasco sauce to the world. Hazard's "Shrewsbury Tomatoketchup" recipe, which was eventually sold to Heinz, was fermented, which explains why ketchup in the mid-1800s was seen as a healthy food. Unfortunately, commercial ketchup is no longer fermented and instead is preserved through chemicals and heat and loaded with high-fructose corn syrup and other refined sweeteners. This story illustrates the glaring difference between tomato ketchup consumption in the past and now; in the past, ketchup contained healthy, fermented ingredients, and the bottles were small, suggesting that people consumed small amounts at any given time. I have developed this recipe in the same spirit. My kids love it, and I feel good serving it to them.

> 2 (6-ounce) cans tomato paste
> ⅓ cup water
> ¼ cup pure maple syrup
> 2 tablespoons brine from lacto-fermented vegetables (such as Amazing Sauerkraut, page 50) or live whey from making Mesophilic Yogurt (page 183)
> 2 tablespoons apple cider vinegar
> 1 tablespoon unsulphured molasses
> ¼ cup unrefined sugar (such as Sucanat or muscovado)
> ¾ teaspoon sea salt
> ¼ teaspoon ground mustard

¼ teaspoon ground cinnamon
⅛ teaspoon ground cloves
⅛ teaspoon ground allspice
Pinch cayenne pepper, or more to taste

Combine all the ingredients in a medium bowl and whisk well. Pour into a pint-size mason jar, cover, and leave on the counter for 2 days to ferment. Use immediately or cover and store in the fridge for up to 6 months.

FERMENTED MUSTARD

We developed this recipe to accompany the sourdough pretzels from our microbakery, Rise. Fermentation boosts the flavor and probiotic content, and the combination of raw honey and unrefined sugar adds a little sweetness to balance the heat of the mustard.

⅓ cup yellow mustard seeds

¼ cup brown mustard seeds

½ cup plus 1 tablespoon raw apple cider vinegar

⅓ cup plus 1 tablespoon water

2 tablespoons brine from lacto-fermented vegetables (such as Amazing Sauerkraut, page 50) or live whey from making Mesophilic Yogurt (page 183)

2 tablespoons raw honey

⅓ cup unrefined sugar (such as Sucanat or muscovado)

Combine the mustard seeds, apple cider vinegar, water, and brine in a small bowl. Stir to combine, cover, and set aside to soak and ferment for 2 days.

Transfer the mixture to a food processor or blender, along with the honey and sugar. Process until most of the seeds have been ground and the mustard is thick. Transfer to a pint-size mason jar. Use immediately or cover and store in the fridge for up to 6 months.

Chapter 4

GRAINS

WHEAT, SOURDOUGH, AND THEIR COUSINS

It was getting late and, honestly, I was beat. As usual, Christina and I had been up all night with Brianna, our older daughter, prepping for the Kent Island Farmer's Market, where Brianna's fledgling sourdough bread business, Rise, had a stand. Every Thursday afternoon, we showed up with hundreds of loaves of bread, baguettes, crackers, pretzels, focaccia, and more — all sourdough — and because we wanted everything as fresh as possible, the night before was always a crush.

The three of us, each working on only a few hours' sleep, had spent the morning baking off the baguettes and pretzels, packing preorders, and loading the pickup truck and Jeep with the tent, two tables, the rest of the setup, and of course the stars of the show: elegant baguettes wrapped in paper, sliced sandwich breads, bakery boxes full of decadent focaccia, artisanal boules and bâtards, piles of crackers, and still-warm-from-the-oven pretzels.

All of it had been selling out quickly, as it always does, and we were nearly done for the day. The constant roar of traffic on Interstate Route 50 next to the shopping center parking lot where the market is located was steadily embedding between my eyes as a dull, thrumming ache. In the early winter evening, the light was falling fast, clear and golden over the Chesapeake Bay just a quarter mile west of us. The crowd was thinning out, and we were beginning to tidy up in preparation for the breakdown when an elderly gentleman hurried toward us, moving as best he could across the uneven macadam with his cane. He wore a ballcap that showed him to be a US Navy veteran.

"Focaccia?" he asked, looking worriedly at our nearly empty display tables. "Don't tell me I'm too late!"

Brianna grinned and reached into a bag behind the table, where she had secreted the last of the rectangular, flaxen-colored loaves flecked with rosemary, olive oil, and Celtic sea salt.

"Hello again," she said, handing it across the table. "We knew you'd want one."

The man clapped his hands together. "Ah, I can't thank you enough! It's the only bread my wife can eat. She loves bread, but if it's not your sourdough, there's hell to pay!"

As they finished their transaction, I felt a little of the day's tiredness lift. How many times had we heard nearly those same words from Brianna's customers? Dozens, at least. All with the same kind of story, and it was a story I knew well. Every time I heard some version of it, I thought about how our relationship with this most fundamental, foundational, and human of foods has become so confusing and contentious. For years, diet gurus have treated bread (and its gluten and carbohydrates) like the spawn of Satan itself. And for years, so did I.

When I was a wrestler in high school and college, all of my coaches advocated a grain-heavy diet that included whole-grain foods and breads but also any foods that would help me carbo-load before a competition. In high school, we held team pasta nights, and when I was on Ohio State's wrestling squad, we regularly descended on a local restaurant for its all-you-can-eat pasta extravaganza. But once I stopped competing, the weight piled on, and I turned to every trendy diet that came down the pike to lose the pounds. Most of them treated carbs—and, of course, bread—as forbidden fruit. I knew there were legitimate health and weight-loss benefits to a low-carb diet, and as with everything I do, I went all in, completely eliminating grains and bread from my kitchen and my plate. Not until my research began to focus on ancestral and traditional food-processing technologies and techniques did I realize two important truths when it comes to grains and bread in our diets: (1) It doesn't have to be all or nothing because (2) it's just not that simple.

Today, my family and I enjoy bread, crackers, pizza, and other grain-based foods, though we always consume them in moderation. With the rare exception of a birthday cake or some special-occasion treat—when the emotional or cultural situation allows for or even requires that special case—we ensure that the grains we consume have been processed in ways that make them as safe and nourishing as possible. When it comes to bread and other baked goods, this means using the traditional sourdough process that relies on a combination of wild bacteria and yeast to produce a long and slow fermentation. By doing this, we approach bread—and the grains from which it's made—as we approach every other food in this book, using processes our ancestors began using nearly 15,000 years ago to make grains safe and to maximize their nutrition. If you were one of the many people who began baking sourdough bread during the Covid-19 pandemic, you, too, were tapping into these traditional techniques. And while for many people the act of pandemic sourdough baking was practical (a traditional sourdough doesn't use commercial yeast, which in many places had become hard to source), rewarding (did you see all those proud photos of fresh-baked loaves on Facebook and Instagram?), and even mentally and emotionally beneficial (there is something peaceful and mindful about the thoughtfulness inherent in bread baking), genuine sourdough is also the most delicious, safe, and nourishing bread you can eat.

The irony is that bread *should* be forbidden fruit, but not because of the reasons you've always been told. Rather, it's because at first glance, grains have no business being in our diets. And here, I'm going to ask you to refine your concept of grains. When we hear that word, most of us think of "amber waves of grain" and interpret that to mean wheat, oats, perhaps rye, even barley. But a grain is simply a seed—in this case, a seed from a type of grass, like wheat—and for the purposes of this discussion, we need to categorize it with other seeds as well, including nuts and legumes. Although they may come from different sources—a peanut, for instance, is a legume that grows as a seed in a pod, while a walnut is a nut (technically it's a drupe) and is the seed of a tree—they all share common, critically important characteristics; and in terms of our health, they all present the same challenges. Simply put, we're not biologically built to safely process them or easily derive nutrition from them.

Seeds have one mission: to survive long enough until the right environmental conditions come along for them to germinate and sprout a new plant. They accomplish this mission with remarkable adaptations. Some nuts, such as walnuts and pecans, have developed hard, durable protective shells. Some seeds, such as maple samaras, have evolved winged seed pods that help carry them through the air to new locations. Others, like burdock, have hooks that latch into an animal's fur for transport. (Fun seed fact: In an inspired case of biomimicry, it was the tenaciously clingy seed of a burdock that prompted the early concept of what we now know as Velcro. Anyone who's ever had a dog come home covered in these burrs knows how stubborn and well-traveled these seeds can be.) In all cases, the most important objective is for the seed to survive the trip, whether the journey is through the digestive tract of an animal or carried miles on the wind. If the seed, nut, or legume germinates too early, it exposes itself, and without the right environment it will die.

Physically, most seeds have a tough, protective outer coating to help them survive long periods of dormancy. Chemically, many seeds and nuts have developed toxins that help them ward off fungi, diseases, and insects. Bitter almonds, less common in American cuisine but used in marzipan, fruitcakes, and syrups in Europe and Asia, contain hydrocyanic acid (or prussic acid), a cousin of cyanide, with all of its potentially dangerous effects. Most nuts and drupes, especially almonds, cashews, and hazelnuts, are very high in oxalates, those same troublesome characters we find in spinach and some other greens. Perhaps most problematic for us, however, is that some of these toxins are antinutrients that hinder the ability of our digestive tracts to assimilate minerals. Among these is phytic acid, a compound found only in plants. As a storage mechanism for phosphorus, it plays an important role in providing a food source for the new plant when it germinates. But from a human health perspective, it's a big problem. Since we humans have one simple stomach chamber, we don't possess the enzyme phytase, which is necessary to break down and deactivate phytic acid. Instead, this antinutrient binds with minerals and essential amino acids in our guts, rendering them inaccessible to us nutritionally.

Lectins are another antinutrient and are found in nuts and legumes, such as beans and peanuts, as well as many grains. For example, a lectin known as phytohemagglutinin occurs in high levels in legumes and beans and is especially high in red kidney beans. According to the US Food and Drug Administration's *Handbook of Foodborne Pathogenic Microorganisms and Natural Toxins* (aka the *Bad Bug Book*), eating even as few as four or five soaked but uncooked (raw) red kidney beans can trigger poisoning symptoms that begin with extreme nausea and vomiting followed by diarrhea and abdominal pain. In addition to being toxic, lectins inhibit our body's ability to make use of calcium, iron, phosphorus, and zinc, and can lead to inflammation. Other antinutrients found in grains, seeds, nuts, and legumes include tannins and saponins. They all affect our body's ability to make use of the food we consume in the safest and most nourishing way possible. When we consume raw, unsoaked, unfermented, unsprouted grains, seeds, and legumes, not only do we deny our bodies the maximum amount of nutrition they have to offer, we let them rob our bodies of the nutrition we are attempting to obtain from other food sources.

Unlike us, some animals have digestive tracts that have evolved to deal with these obstacles, and it's worth examining how they process seeds and grains, because our ancestors learned to mimic these processes outside their bodies, and we should do the same. For example, most birds are granivorous, subsisting primarily on seeds and grain. Near the beginning of their digestive tract they have a crop—an enlarged muscular pouch—where grains and seeds can be held for up to 16 hours. In this warm, moist environment, seeds absorb moisture, ferment, and, depending on the amount of time they remain in the crop, can even begin to sprout. These chemical processes work to neutralize the phytic acid and other chemicals, break down complex carbohydrates into simple sugars, and lower the pH, transforming a difficult-to-digest grain into something the bird's body can safely and more effectively use. Next, these partially processed grains travel to the gizzard. Here, small stones—called gastroliths, which the birds intentionally consume—work with a pair of powerful muscular disks to mechanically break down and grind the seeds and grains. Given the complexity of these biological processes, you can imagine what might happen to a bird if grains bypassed the crop and gizzard and went straight to the stomach. Yet that's effectively what we are doing when we eat the majority of the bread that's in our grocery stores. Inadequate processing of these foods may account for many people's increasing intolerance to gluten. On the other hand, we can mimic what happens inside the crop and gizzard — soaking, slow and long fermentation, sometimes sprouting, and grinding — outside our bodies and then consume grains in a state that can deliver safe, available nutrition.

So, while it's biologically accurate to say that we have no real business eating grains, seeds, legumes, and even nuts (and, by extension, bread), rejecting them wholesale isn't the only answer. Nor should it be, since these foods have health benefits that are worth the effort. Instead, we need to approach them like every other food we talk about in this book, by using techniques to make them as safe and nutritious as possible. The easiest way for humans to make grains and seeds more nutritious and easier to digest is by fooling them into letting down their defenses by mimicking the warm, moist conditions that prompt them to germinate. Various techniques that our ancestors developed, such as soaking, sprouting, fermenting, nixtamalizing (more on this later), grinding, and cooking, radically alter the chemical and physical composition of grains and seeds, making them more nutritious and digestible.

It may come as a surprise, but some archaeologists believe that one of the first complex processing technologies that enabled our ancestors of some 13,000 years ago to derive nutrition from grain was brewing beer. This process required grains such as barley to be soaked until they sprouted (known in modern brewing as malting), disabling antinutrients like phytic acid and activating the amylase enzyme, which is responsible for the crucial conversion from complex carbohydrates into fermentable and digestible sugars. Beermakers would halt the conversion process by drying and sometimes roasting the sprouted grains, which could be stored for long periods of time. Later, the grains were heated to a specific temperature and held there to complete the conversion of carbohydrates to sugars. The nutrients released from the grain during this process were then collected in the form of wort, which was boiled, cooled, and then fermented. We rarely think of beer as a source of nutrition, but beer-making was a food technology milestone for our ancestors, who used it to extract easily digestible nutrition from otherwise nutritionally inaccessible seeds. It's important to note that until the 19th century, just as with sourdough bread, beer-making employed a fermentation of bacteria and yeast. Unfortunately, just like bread, most beer today is made with just yeast—and commercial yeast at that—although there is a niche but growing market for "sour" beers made through bacteria and yeast fermentation. And the good thing about beer is that no matter how it is fermented, many of the grains are sprouted/malted in the early stages of the process.

Our own saliva is another source of the amylase enzyme, and some cultures chew and spit out the grains as the first step in the brewing process. Not only does this soften and mechanically break down the grains, it allows the amylase enzymes in the saliva to begin the conversion of complex carbohydrates before the grains are fermented to make alcohol. Chicha—an ancient, corn-based, fermented beverage based in Mesoamerica—is made through this process in traditional households today. In Japan, a form of sake known as kuchikamizake (which translates to "mouth chew sake") was traditionally made from the spit of virgin girls. In the rainforest of Peru, a local alcoholic drink, masato, is made from chewing and spitting the yuca root. It's entirely plausible that our ancestors employed this method.

Along with brewing beer, baking bread also became a way for our ancestors to consume grains. Early farmers had one up on us nutritionally from the start, because the grains they grew contained many more nutrients than most of what's available to us today. (Recall that statistic from Chapter 2: USDA researchers found that in 14 varieties of wheat grown between 1873 and 2000, when the average per-acre harvest more than tripled, the wheat's micronutrient content declined dramatically—for example, 28 percent less iron, 34 percent less zinc, and 36 percent less selenium over the period.) After they harvested the grains, they dried and stored them. But storage facilities then, as you can imagine, weren't exactly climate controlled. A combination of pervious storage and incomplete drying resulted in moisture, which encouraged the grains to sprout. No doubt this frustrated our farmer forebears, who wanted the grains to stay dry and intact for long-term storage, but it benefited them nutritionally by essentially predigesting the grain outside their bodies and beginning that important complex-carbohydrate conversion. Next came grinding on stones (remember the birds' gastroliths?). Then, they mixed the grain with water and salt and let it slowly ferment in the presence of both wild bacteria and yeast through the addition of a carefully maintained mother culture. After a long fermentation process that sometimes lasted for days, the loaf was formed and finally baked.

In all of these examples, the process began with soaking and/or sprouting the grains, and this ancient technique remains eminently doable and valuable today. Since we don't have the ability to metabolize phytic acid, reducing a food's phytic acid content is a logical way to help our bodies better absorb important minerals. When it comes to grains, seeds, and legumes, sprouting and soaking can help accomplish this. Sprouting has been shown to reduce the phytic acid content in grains by up to 40 percent, while a 2012 study found that soaking chickpeas (another legume) for 12 hours decreased it by up to almost 56 percent. Sprouting has also been shown to make protein more soluble and digestible in millet (by 55 percent) and barley (by 80 percent) as well as to increase vitamins such as folate, niacin, riboflavin, thiamin, vitamin A, and vitamin C. For example, a 2007 study reports that after wheat was sprouted for 4.5 days, the B vitamin folate increased by 3.5 times. Sprouting also affects the levels of gluten. One study on sprouting several varieties of wheat over eight days found total gluten reduced by 35 percent in kamut wheat and 62 percent in svevo wheat. Even more significant, though, was the reduction in the type of gluten that provokes autoimmune responses, as in celiac disease. The reduction of toxic gluten ranged from 30 percent with kamut to 79 percent with svevo.

But sprouting is just one ancient technique that's beneficial when dealing with grains. Even more important is long, slow bacterial fermentation, which our ancestors employed when they made beer and bread. This process, when used to make sourdough, remains the gold standard for transforming grains into their most digestible, delicious, fulfilling, and nutritious form. Genuine sourdough bread is more nutritious than even homemade white, whole wheat, rye, or oat bread because fermentation makes the grains' vitamins and minerals more accessible to our bodies. As a tool to remove phytic acid, fermentation is highly effective; studies on brown rice indicate that fermentation decreased phytic acid content between 56 and 96 percent, and when pearl millet was both sprouted and fermented, phytate dropped by 88.3 percent. Sourdough is easier to digest because it has already started to break down chemically and physically, essentially being predigested outside our bodies. The sourdough process lowers the glycemic index (GI), the rating system that indicates how quickly a food raises your blood sugar on a scale from 1 to 100 (100 is pure glucose). This means that eating sourdough bread is a completely different experience for your body (and your blood sugar) than eating modern commercial bread; in effect, your body treats sourdough bread more like a vegetable than a carbohydrate. For example, according to a study published in 2020 in the journal *Aging Clinical and Experimental Research,* 30 grams of white wheat or whole wheat bread has a GI of 71, while the same serving of sourdough bread rates at 54. High-GI foods are classified at being over 70, and low-GI foods are classified as being under 55. This means that the sourdough process *itself* is responsible for moving bread from a high to low GI category, regardless of whether the bread is made from white or whole wheat flour. To put this in perspective, a yam has a GI rating of 54, a parsnip 52, and green peas 51. Early studies even show promise that sourdough fermentation can degrade gluten enough to make it nontoxic for people with celiac disease.

In addition to being more nourishing, genuine sourdough is a symphony of texture and flavor truly born of local terroir, thanks to the dependence on wild bacteria and yeasts that exist all around us—in the air we breathe, on our skin, on our kitchen counters, and in our grains and food. When we start and maintain a sourdough mother culture, we are simply harnessing the hyperlocal bacteria and yeasts specific to our microenvironment. Studies have traced sourdough bread not just to the geographic region it came from, or even the bakery in which it was made, but to the actual baker's hands that traded bacteria and yeasts with the dough. Our culture tends to associate bacteria with illness, but this, like so many other narrowed perceptions, requires rethinking. Wild bacteria are hugely beneficial, and the idea that we can exploit them in the foods we make is a profound connection to the natural world around us and the terroir that defines and characterizes our culinary environments.

A word about my use of the word *genuine* when talking about sourdough: The term *sourdough* has no official or legal standing, so we can't use it alone to provide guidance on purchasing bread. Companies take shortcuts and use lactic acid or something similar to produce a quickly risen, yeasted bread that artificially tastes like genuine sourdough. Truly genuine sourdough bread contains three ingredients: flour, water, and salt. If any ingredients on the label sound like lactic, citric, ascorbic, or acetic acid (vinegar), it's not true long-fermented bread, and you might as well eat a loaf of Wonder Bread, nutritionally speaking.

Some people think that making sourdough is too time-consuming and complicated. I used to think so as well. In fact, when I first started experimenting with sourdough, I allowed the process to control my schedule. For years, I carried fermenting dough around with me, especially on the weekends, so that I could tend to it while continuing to engage in my busy family's activities and running errands. I can even remember interrupting a lovely restaurant date with my wife as my iPhone alarm sounded, reminding me it was time to go outside and tend to the dough that was sitting in a tub in our car. Over time, however, this became too much even for me, so I can only imagine how few readers would want to do the same.

But here's what I did: I learned how to manipulate temperature and hydration and make my refrigerator do most of the work. In fact, much to everyone's relief, I haven't carried dough around in years, relying instead on the refrigerator to slow down fermentation. So, while the sourdough breadmaking process can take upwards of a day and a half, it requires only a total of 20 minutes of my input, in small chunks, interspersed with longer periods during which billions of beneficial microorganisms do the heavy lifting. People also think that sourdough automatically means bread, but any baked good can be sourdough—cinnamon buns, croissants, pie crusts, pancakes, and more. And the process can be controlled, so these won't taste sour. As the baker, you can manage a variety of factors—including time, temperature, and amount of water—to influence flavor and sourness.

And while the issue of gluten intolerance is complex (and celiac disease something else entirely), I can say from personal experience that as long as I eat breads and other wheat-based products—in moderation—that are put through the bacterial fermentation sourdough process, I feel fine. Anything else still wreaks havoc on my gut and results in inflammation and other unpleasant health problems. Likewise, many of the people who buy our daughter's sourdough breads and other products tell us that while they can't tolerate other wheat-based breads, they can eat her sourdough without any adverse effects. It's not simply the presence of gluten that is the issue, but rather how the gluten has been processed; the bacterial fermentation process chemically and physically transforms the gluten into something safer and more digestible.

Long-fermented sourdough is a brilliant and ages-old solution for transforming the seeds we know as grain. But what about other members of our seed category, including nuts, actual seeds, and legumes? As we saw earlier with red kidney beans, legumes can also be problematic when it comes to toxins and antinutrients. The only way to make red kidney beans safe for human consumption is through a combination of soaking and cooking; soaking in a slightly alkaline solution maximizes the detoxification. A 2008 study published in *Nutrition and Food Science* reported a 78 percent reduction in phytic acid and 66 percent in tannin by soaking red kidney beans in water with baking soda and then cooking them. Nuts and seeds, though, are more problematic. They're valuable sources of protein, especially for people who follow a plant-based diet. But while they do contain protein and other nourishment, it comes at a cost. In addition to many of the antinutrients and toxins other grains possess, many nuts and seeds are extremely high in oxalates, a particularly dangerous toxin that builds up in our bodies over time. According to Healthline.com, most healthcare providers suggest limiting oxalate intake to less than 40 to 50 milligrams per day. Consider, then, that 100 grams of roasted almonds contains 469 milligrams of oxalates, roasted cashews contain 262, and raw hazelnuts contain 222. Sesame and poppy seeds are also high in oxalates.

Then there's the manner in which we eat nuts. When we mistakenly believe that nuts and seeds are nutritional powerhouses that are entirely safe to consume, we think, "If some is good, more must be better." Nuts, seeds, and food products made from them become go-to ingredients in our recipes and snacks in our diets. Milks made from them become staples in households that reject the modern dairy industry and seek a healthier diet, yet consumption of almond milk is now producing kidney stones in children. Baked goods made from nut flours (such as almond flour) become gluten-free alternatives. This really is a ticking time bomb in our pantries and refrigerators, and whether soaking and sprouting can ameliorate some of these issues is up for debate. The fact is, not enough formal research has been done to explore detoxification of nuts and seeds, although there is some promise in fermentation and eating nuts along with supplements such as calcium and magnesium. The few studies that do exist refute soaking and sprouting as viable detoxification strategies. Soaking nuts, despite the lay literature, does not seem to make any difference in the phytate or oxalate content, and more research must be done. Nor does roasting seem to detoxify nuts or make them more bioavailable, although it does release flavors and aromas. Studies suggest that in certain situations, roasting can also reduce oxidative stress, making the fat in nuts less likely to go rancid. Bottom line in our household is this: We don't really trust nuts. We eat very few, and we are highly selective about those we do eat.

This category of foods — grains, nuts, and legumes — we depend on so thoroughly is far more complicated than it looks, and there's a great deal of misinformation and even lore about these foods that muddies things even more. We need to adopt the soundest, most proven and reliable strategies for processing them, as well as moderating our consumption. But as with all foods that our forebears learned how to process to gain the greatest and safest nutrition, simply excluding them is neither sustainable nor necessary. Few things are as comforting as a slice of fresh bread, warm from the oven, rich with tradition, flavor, texture, and terroir, shared with the people you love. Not everyone will want to accept bread back into the fold. But for those who do want to include bread and grains in their diet, baking genuine sourdough is the healthiest way to do it. It's fun, it's empowering, and it's easier than you think.

TIPS AND RECIPES

GRAINS GO OR NO-GO

I devised this list to consider the biological and cultural components of deciding what to eat when it comes to grain-based foods. Here's how it works: To decide whether to eat a food containing grain, see if you can answer yes to the first three questions. Yes answers to each subsequent question help build the case for eating it. Certainly, in the real world at any given moment, the decision is more organic and fluid, but this list helps illustrate the decision-making process:

1. Does eating the food provide me with any important nutrients, either because of the grains it contains or because of other ingredients?
2. Will I derive pleasure from eating this food?
3. Are there cultural reasons why eating this food at this particular moment makes sense?
4. Is it homemade, made from scratch, or made by someone who cares about what my family and I put in our bodies?
5. Have the grains been processed in some way to increase the nutrient density, accessibility, and/or digestibility, such as through fermentation, soaking, and sprouting?
6. Have the grains been processed using more than one of the strategies above?
7. Are the grains high-quality/organic?

8. Are the grains whole?
9. Are the grains ancient or heritage?

Thinking in this new way has significantly improved my family's approach to grains. First, and perhaps most important, there is much less guilt and fear about eating certain foods in my house. It is OK—in fact, it's expected—to eat a piece of birthday cake; the social repercussions of not doing so far outweigh the "healthier" choice of resisting, purely because of the joy that it brings the maker and the recipient of the cake. Second, this approach also lets me use grains as what I call blank slates to support a whole host of nutritious and delicious foods, such as quiche, risotto, pizza, and pasta. When combined with everything from eggs to a diverse range of vegetables, meats, fats, and cheeses, these grains create foods that are delicious and nutritious, and transform an otherwise overly restrictive dinner table to one that is vibrant, diverse, accessible, and healthier.

DETOXIFICATION STRATEGIES: BEST PRACTICES

Grains: A combination of sprouting and bacterial fermentation is the best, followed by only bacterial fermentation, followed by only sprouting. From here, a less effective but still useful method is simply soaking in an acid solution such as kefir, or water mixed with lemon juice or vinegar. The best bread you can make is a bacterial-fermented sourdough bread made with sprouted grain flour (although this flour is expensive), followed by sourdough made with non-sprouted flour. You can use any flour to make sourdough, including wheat, rye, einkorn, spelt, or even gluten-free flours.

Legumes: A combination of soaking with baking soda followed by cooking (ideally using a pressure cooker) is the best option. Soybeans are particularly toxic and should be avoided unless fermented and, even then, consumed in moderation.

Seeds: Select seeds with lower oxalate content such as sunflower, pumpkin, watermelon, and flax seeds, while staying away from high-oxalate-content seeds, such as sesame seeds and poppy seeds. Sprouting is the best thing to do with them, followed by soaking. Simply roasting them to improve flavor and shelf life is the third-best approach.

Nuts: Select nuts with lower oxalate and other tannin content. I avoid almonds, cashews, Brazil nuts, and pine nuts, as well as products made from them, including all nut "milks." Whatever your choice, it is best to eat nuts in moderation.

SPROUTING GRAINS

Obtain high-quality, preferably organic whole grains that have not been processed in a way that would prohibit them from sprouting. They need the hull and germ, bran, and endosperm. Pearled, parched, split, rolled, or chopped grains will not work. In other words, the grains must be dormant, but alive. Sprouted grains can used as toppings on dishes such as salad and are fantastic when incorporated into dough for Airfield Sourdough Bread (see page 135).

Place the grains in a large jar. Do not fill more than one-third of the jar, as the grains will expand to approximately three times their original size.

Secure a layer of cheesecloth or porous material around the rim with a rubber band or other fastener. You need something that is porous enough to allow water to pass through, but fine enough to keep the grains behind.

Fill the jar with warm water, swirl to mix, then strain out the water. Fill the jar once again with warm water, leaving about 1 inch of headspace. Allow the grains to soak overnight to prepare them for sprouting.

The next day, invert the jar, drain the grains, refill with warm water, swirl to mix, invert again to drain, and prop the jar upside down at an angle in a bowl so it continues to drain.

Continue to rinse and drain twice a day until the sprouts are between ⅛ and ¼ inch long. It should take anywhere from one to five days depending on the grain and the temperature of the room. We want to fool the grains into letting down their defenses, to deactivate the phytic acid, start to convert the complex carbohydrates, and begin to sprout. However, we want to stop the process at the ideal point — the point at which the grain is safe and digestible, but before it puts too much energy into the production of new life.

At this point the grains can be used right away, or stored in an airtight container in the refrigerator for up to 1 week or in the freezer for up to 6 months.

SOAKING GRAINS

Ideally, grains should be sprouted. However, once they have been pearled, rolled, cracked, or ground, they no longer possess the ability to sprout. The next best choice is to soak them, a simple process that still accomplishes many (though not all) of the benefits of fermenting and/or sprouting. It is worth the minimal added effort of quickly mixing together a few ingredients and letting them sit on the counter.

The typical overnight soak includes warm water and the addition of something acidic; the slight acidity helps neutralize the phytic acid in the grains and keep the mixture safe from harmful pathogens. Ideal choices for the acidic addition are live whey, yogurt, clabber, kefir, or raw vinegar. Pasteurized vinegar or lemon juice will work too, but they're not teeming with the live probiotics that are present in the other options. I use a ratio of 1 tablespoon of something acidic to 1 cup of water. The basic technique is as follows:

1. Place your grains in a glass or ceramic container and cover with a mixture of warm water and acidic medium of your choice, maintaining the ratio of 1 tablespoon acid to 1 cup water. Make sure your volume of water is three times the volume of grains, because the grains will expand as they absorb the moisture.
2. Cover the container and let it sit on the counter for at least 8 hours, or overnight. Drain if necessary, then use right away, refrigerate for up to 1 week, or freeze for up to 6 months.

SOAKED OVERNIGHT OATS

SERVES 4

A slight variation on the basic technique for soaking grains can produce a convenient, delicious, nutrient-dense breakfast. Prepare a batch of overnight oats whenever you have a chance and store them in the refrigerator for a no-hassle breakfast or snack.

> 1½ cups rolled oats (preferably sprouted, see page 118)
> 1½ cups kefir, raw milk clabber, or yogurt
> 3 tablespoons pure maple syrup, raw honey, or unrefined sugar
>   (such as Sucanat or muscovado)
> 2 tablespoons unsweetened shredded coconut
> ¾ teaspoon pure vanilla extract
> Pinch sea salt

In a medium bowl, mix all the ingredients. Pack the mixture into four glass jars and cover. Place the jars on the counter or in a cabinet at room temperature for 6 to 8 hours. The soaked oats can be eaten immediately or transferred to the refrigerator for a few days. These are delicious cold, so an ideal schedule would be to mix this up before you go to work in the morning, let it sit on the counter during the day, and transfer it to the fridge when you return home from work at the end of the day. That way, they are ready to go when you wake up in the morning.

Note:

If using "porridge" oats, add an additional ¾ cup kefir, milk clabber, or yogurt, because they absorb more moisture.

What to do with leftovers?

Dehydrate them! Spread out the leftover oat mixture on a parchment-lined rimmed baking sheet and place in your oven at its lowest setting (for most of us that is 170°F) for several hours, until fully dehydrated and brittle. Remove from the oven, break into smaller pieces, and store in an airtight container at room temperature for up to 3 months. There are numerous ways you can use these dried, soaked, sweetened oats, including as a base for Cricket Granola (page 219).

For Chocolate Overnight Oats:

To the above master recipe, add 4½ tablespoons unsweetened cocoa powder and omit the vanilla.

For Citrus Overnight Oats:

To the above master recipe, add the grated zest and juice of 1 lemon, lime, or orange.

For Hot Porridge:

Make the overnight oats as in the master recipe, but instead of eating them cold, add ½ cup milk and warm them in a small saucepan over medium heat, stirring occasionally, until heated through and the liquid is absorbed to the desired consistency.

COOKING BEANS AND CHICKPEAS

MAKES ABOUT 6 CUPS

When we soak beans or chickpeas overnight in an alkaline solution created by adding baking soda to water, the final product is as safe and nourishing as possible. In much the same way that nixtamalization does with maize (see Chapter 5), this process detoxifies the antinutrients in the chickpeas and makes the nutrients more bioavailable. Soaking in an alkaline solution also reduces the cooking time and improves the texture by breaking down the pectin more quickly and thoroughly.

> 2 teaspoons baking soda
>
> 4 cups water
>
> 2 cups dry beans or chickpeas
>
> 1 onion, halved
>
> 2 garlic cloves, peeled

Combine the baking soda and water in a large bowl and stir to dissolve. Add the beans or chickpeas and cover the bowl. Soak for at least 12 hours or up to 24 hours.

Drain the beans or chickpeas in a colander, rinse well, and transfer to a medium pot. Add the onion, garlic, and enough water to cover by at least 2 inches. Bring to a boil over medium-high heat, then reduce to a simmer and cover. Cook until soft. This may take 1 to 3 hours, depending on the variety, size, and age of the beans, as well as the humidity in your kitchen. Add water as needed to ensure that the beans are always covered with water. Alternatively, cook the beans with enough water to cover, the onion, and garlic cloves in a pressure cooker for 30 to 40 minutes.

If you plan on using the chickpeas to make Avi's Traditional Hummus (page 123) or the beans to make Refried Beans (page 125), it is critical for them to be very soft—they should crush easily when pressed between your fingers.

AVI'S TRADITIONAL HUMMUS

SERVES 4 TO 6

This recipe was shared with me by my friend, the Israeli chef Avi Mor Mosseri, whom I met at the Italian Culinary Institute. Avi was the first chef to introduce me to the advantages of adding baking soda to the soaking water for beans. This is hands down the best hummus recipe I have ever found. The tahini paste (made from sesame seeds) has been replaced by sunflower butter to drastically reduce the oxalate content in the hummus.

Avi explained to me that dry chickpeas oxidize and deteriorate very quickly when cooked, and even more quickly when mashed to a paste. This is why hummus is best when served warm, right after preparation. It may be kept cold for only one more day. Serious hummus restaurants in the Middle East prepare it fresh to serve, and many of them cook the daily portion of the chickpeas for the day's sale and close the shop when sold and finished. This is why a truly good hummus is hard to get anywhere — so why not simply make it at home?

> 2 cups soaked and cooked chickpeas, drained when still warm (see page 122)
> ½ cooked onion from cooking the chickpeas
> 1 garlic clove, peeled
> 1 tablespoon olive oil, plus more for drizzling
> 1 teaspoon freshly squeezed lemon juice
> ½ cup sunflower butter
> 1 cup warm water, as necessary
> Sea salt and freshly ground black pepper
> Finely chopped fresh parsley, for garnish
> Butter Bite Crackers (page 133), for serving

Combine the chickpeas, onion, garlic, olive oil, and lemon juice in a food processor and process until very smooth. Add the sunflower butter and process until smooth. If the paste is too thick, add the warm water, 1 tablespoon at a time, processing in between additions, until the desired consistency is reached. The hummus should be stable and not liquidy; if it turns too liquidy, balance it by adding more sunflower butter. Season with salt and pepper to taste.

Serve warm, topped with a drizzle of extra virgin olive oil and some finely chopped parsley, along with crackers for spreading.

REFRIED BEANS

SERVES 4 TO 6

Unfortunately, most cans of refried beans contain nothing more than mashed cooked beans. This tasteless version of a delicious and nourishing traditional food has succumbed to the low-fat craze over the past few decades and is even sold as a low-fat food. The reality is that traditionally, refried beans were cooked, then "refried" with lard, which boosted the nutrition, flavor, and aroma. The key to creating the most delicious, safe, and nourishing refried beans is the combination of soaking the beans in an alkaline solution, discarding the cooking water (most refried beans recipes keep it and add some back in), and cooking with high-quality lard you either rendered yourself or sourced from a reliable producer.

1 cup lard, butter, or bacon grease
6 cups soaked and cooked pinto or black beans, drained
    (see page 122)
Sea salt and freshly ground black pepper
1 cup warm Trash Bone Broth (page 79) or water (optional)

Heat the lard in a large skillet over medium-high heat until it is melted and hot. Add the beans and mash them with a potato masher or spoon. Continue to cook and stir until all of the lard has been incorporated into the beans. Remove from the heat and season with salt and pepper to taste. I like my refried beans thick and chunky, but if you prefer a thinner consistency, add a little warm bone broth or water, 1 tablespoon at a time, stirring until the desired consistency is reached. To achieve smoother refried beans, further process them with a stick blender directly in the pan, or transfer to a food processor and process until smooth. Serve warm.

SOURDOUGH

THE STAND MIXER AND SCALE

The recipes that follow are primarily written for someone using a kitchen scale to measure and a stand mixer to mix. Both tools help a great deal in achieving a consistent final product; reducing as many variables as possible is one of the best ways to become skilled as quickly as possible. However, you can still make these recipes without these two tools. I have provided volume measurements if you don't have a scale (just disregard the references to scaling ingredients) and included instructions if you don't have a stand mixer.

THE DANISH DOUGH WHISK

You can use a spoon or spatula to mix sourdough, but it can be difficult, especially for refreshing the mother culture. The stiff, sticky dough clings to the surface, making it hard to clean, and it can feel like you are pushing around concrete. For less than $10, the best tool for this is a Danish dough whisk. It has a stiff, irregular, open wire structure that easily and efficiently mixes the dough.

BACK IT UP!

Once you have established your sourdough mother, you should create a backup culture in case something ever happens to the original. Simply take about 100 grams of your original mother culture, spread it out thin on a piece of parchment paper, and allow it to fully dry at room temperature. Do *not* use a stove; you do not want to kill the bacteria and yeast. Once it is dry, break it into smaller pieces and store it in an airtight container at room temperature indefinitely. It can be reactivated with water and, after a few feedings, will be fully activated and ready for baking.

MOTHER "FLOUR"

If you find yourself with an ample amount of leftover sourdough mother, spread it out on a piece of parchment in as thin a layer as possible and allow it to fully dry at room temperature. Do *not* use a stove; you do not want to kill the bacteria and yeast. Once it is dry, break it up and return it to a flour consistency in a blender or food processor. This "flour" is incredibly valuable, as it has been through the sourdough process and is transformed into its safest and healthiest form. Use as is for bench flour to keep dough from sticking while making bread or to dredge food in before dipping in sourdough batter to help it stick.

KEEPING DOUGH FROM STICKING

There are three ways to keep dough from sticking to your hands and other surfaces: flour, water, and fat. All have their place in different stages of various bread recipes. Here are a few guidelines:

Flour: Any type of flour can be used to keep the dough from sticking during the pre-shaping, bench-resting, shaping, and proofing stages. Make sure to use as little as possible, as this flour will not have been through the sourdough process. I keep a bowl of flour on the side of my workstation for this purpose. Use rice flour to dust the proofing baskets to achieve the best release.

Water: Always keep a container full of water nearby so that you can dip bowl scrapers and spatulas in before transferring dough. Dipping your hands in water during the folding stages is the best way to prevent sticking.

Fat: Fat in the form of lard, butter, or monounsaturated oil (like extra virgin olive oil) is used to grease the container before bulk fermentation to prevent sticking during folding, and in baking pans when making focaccia and sandwich bread to ensure the finished loaf releases after baking. Make sure to stay away from industrial nut and seed oils.

CREATING A SOURDOUGH MOTHER CULTURE

Theoretically, you should only have to start a sourdough mother culture from scratch once in your life. In fact, there are sourdough mother cultures still in use that are more than 150 years old! Once it is established, follow the maintenance schedule below to keep it alive and strong. Be sure to use organic flour and non-chlorinated water to get your sourdough mother started. I recommend using bottled spring water. This is the only time working with sourdough when you must be attentive to the water type you are using. From here on out, tap water is fine, but for the mother culture, you must have non-chlorinated water, and since many public water supplies and even private filter systems introduce chlorine, it's best to use spring water in this application.

Day 1: Mix 45 grams (¼ cup) organic whole wheat flour, 5 grams (2 teaspoons) organic rye flour, and 40 grams (3 tablespoons) non-chlorinated water in a small bowl, loosely cover, and set in a warm location.

Day 2: Mix another 45 grams (¼ cup) organic whole wheat flour, 5 grams (2 teaspoons) organic rye flour, and 40 grams (3 tablespoons) non-chlorinated water in a small bowl, and add to the previous day's mixture. Mix together. Loosely cover and set in a warm location.

Day 3: Mix 100 grams (½ cup) organic whole wheat flour and 80 grams (⅓ cup) non-chlorinated water in a small bowl, and add to the previous day's mixture. Mix together. Loosely cover and set in a warm location.

Day 4: You should have a bubbling, active culture ready for baking. If not, repeat step 3 until you do. Once active, your sourdough mother culture is ready for baking, or you can transfer it to a jar, cover, and store in the fridge for up to 1 week before refreshing.

MAINTAINING A SOURDOUGH MOTHER CULTURE

This recipe is for maintaining a sourdough mother with 80 percent hydration. Each time you refresh your mother culture, it will take between

12 and 16 hours to mature to the point when it is ready to leaven bread using the process outlined below. Follow these steps to maintain your mother so it is always ready each time you bake:

1. About 12 hours before you want to bake, remove the jar of mature mother culture from the fridge.
2. In a medium bowl, mix 200 grams (¾ cup plus 2 tablespoons) 75°F water (at this point, tap water is fine since the culture is already established), 50 grams (¼ cup) mature mother culture, and 250 grams (1⅔ cups) bread flour.
3. Transfer the mixture to a clean jar, cover loosely, and let it ferment at room temperature for 12 to 16 hours. After this period, it is ready to use immediately, or it can be stored in the refrigerator and used anytime up to a week before it needs to be refreshed.

This schedule allows you the freedom to use the culture at a moment's notice. Use the leftover sourdough mother culture for Sourdough Pancakes and Waffles (page 130), Butter Bite Crackers (page 133), or in other recipes. If you let it go long enough that a grayish, acetic-smelling and -tasting liquid (hooch) appears on the surface, pour the liquid off. Don't worry, chances are the mother culture isn't dead. It just needs a little TLC to nurse it back to life. At this stage, it may require refreshing several times to get the culture back to full strength and optimum flavor.

SOURDOUGH PANCAKES AND WAFFLES

This simple recipe produces gorgeous, delicious, and nourishing pancakes. Working with the sourdough mother culture can seem overwhelming at first, but the steps below will help you transform that sticky mass of developed gluten into an amazing pancake batter that everyone will enjoy. It is important to incorporate kefir or other high-quality (preferably live) dairy into the mother to reach the desired consistency at the very beginning of the process. The amount of liquid needed depends on several factors, so I leave it up to you to judge on a case-by-case basis. I am confident this will become a weekly go-to recipe in your house! See the note below for waffle instructions.

450 grams (2 cups) mature sourdough mother culture
   (see page 128)
Kefir, buttermilk, or milk, as needed
1 teaspoon baking powder
½ teaspoon baking soda
½ teaspoon sea salt
1 large egg
2 tablespoons pure maple syrup, raw honey, or sweetener of
   choice, plus more for optional topping
2 tablespoons butter, melted, plus more for the griddle
Fresh blueberries or a few pieces of high-quality dark chocolate
   (optional)
Yogurt, berry sauce, or Fermented Butter (page 189), for topping
   (optional)

Using a moistened spatula, scoop the sourdough mother into a medium bowl and return the rest to the refrigerator. Add kefir (or other liquid)

¼ cup at a time and whisk until a slightly thick batter consistency is achieved. (Using a Danish dough whisk will yield the best results, but a hand mixer or wooden spoon will work just fine.) The consistency of the sourdough mother changes over time, so the amount of liquid you need will vary depending on the age of the mother.

In a small bowl, combine the baking powder, baking soda, and salt. In a separate small bowl, whisk the egg. Add the maple syrup and melted butter to the egg and whisk until the ingredients are combined. Empty the contents of both small bowls into the bowl containing the sourdough mother. Use a wooden spoon to combine.

Warm a griddle or skillet over medium-high heat. Add a pat of butter to the pan, allow it to melt, and swirl the pan to coat the bottom with butter. Use a measuring cup or ladle to transfer the batter to the griddle and use the bottom of the ladle to spread the batter evenly into a circle. Now is the time to add berries or chocolate pieces, if you are using them. Place them one by one directly where you want them and give each one a gentle push into the pancake so they are not sitting on top. (This works better than adding them to the batter, because it lets you make different types of pancakes from the same batch and ensures even distribution of ingredients.) Cook until bubbles begin to form and the edges begin to change color and firm up. Sourdough pancakes will not brown the same way that most pancakes do. They rely on the butter browning to add that special look and texture we all enjoy. Use the spatula to gently lift one side of the pancake to make sure it is browned to your liking. Once ready, flip and begin cooking on the other side. Serve warm with your topping(s) of choice.

Note:

If you are making waffles, increase the melted butter from 2 tablespoons to 3 tablespoons. Follow the manufacturer's directions on your waffle maker to cook the waffles.

SOURDOUGH "TEMPURA" BATTER FOR DEEP FRYING

MAKES ABOUT 1 QUART

By replacing the liquid in the pancake recipe with beer and eliminating the maple syrup and butter, you can make a healthy batter for deep-frying everything from onion rings to fish.

> 450 grams (2 cups) mature sourdough mother culture
> (see page 128)
> 1 (12-ounce) can or bottle beer
> 1 teaspoon baking powder
> ½ teaspoon baking soda
> ½ teaspoon sea salt
> 1 large egg

Using a moistened spatula, scoop the sourdough mother into a medium bowl and return the rest to the refrigerator. Add the beer ¼ cup at a time and whisk until a slightly thin batter consistency is achieved. (A Danish dough whisk will yield the best results, but a hand mixer or wooden spoon will work just fine.) The consistency of the sourdough mother changes over time, so the amount of beer you need will vary depending on the age of the mother.

In a small bowl, combine the baking powder, baking soda, and salt. In a separate small bowl, whisk the egg. Empty the contents of both small bowls into the bowl containing the sourdough mother. Use a wooden spoon to combine.

To ensure the batter sticks, first dredge whatever you are frying in Mother "Flour" (see page 127) or sprouted flour, then dip in batter and deep-fry according to the recipe.

BUTTER BITE CRACKERS

These crackers are one of Rise's top sellers and are an excellent way to transform leftover sourdough mother into a nutritious food with a long shelf life. They look and taste like healthy Wheat Thins and are a perfect complement to cheese or as a snack themselves. The crystalline structure of Maldon sea salt makes it perfect for topping crackers both visually and for how it feels in your mouth when you eat it. Or, for something completely different, replace the salt with everything bagel seasoning to create a cracker that is delectable when topped with cream cheese!

450 grams (2 cups) mature sourdough mother culture
(see page 128)
221 grams (1⅓ cups) whole wheat flour
9 grams (1½ teaspoons) sea salt
66 grams (⅓ cup) unsalted butter, room temperature, plus more,
melted, for brushing
Maldon salt

Combine the sourdough mother, whole wheat flour, salt, and softened butter in the bowl of a stand mixer fitted with the dough hook and mix on speed 1 until all ingredients are fully incorporated. Or, if mixing by hand, stir with a Danish dough whisk or wooden spoon to combine the ingredients until it becomes too difficult to continue. Turn out the dough onto a clean work surface and knead just until all the ingredients are fully incorporated. Transfer the dough to an airtight container or wrap in plastic wrap and refrigerate for 6 to 12 hours to slowly ferment.

Preheat the oven to 350°F. Line several rimmed baking sheets with parchment paper.

Roll the dough into thin sheets (approximately ¹⁄₁₆ inch thick) with a rolling pin or pasta machine. Carefully transfer the dough sheets to the prepared baking sheets, cut into 1½-inch squares, brush the tops with melted butter, and sprinkle with Maldon salt. Bake for 20 to 25 minutes, until crisp and slightly browned. Transfer to a wire rack to cool. When completely cool, store in an airtight container at room temperature, up to several weeks.

AIRFIELD SOURDOUGH BREAD

MAKES 2 LOAVES (OR 12 BUNS)

I developed this formula while my family and I lived in a quaint cottage in Airfield Estates, an educational and working farm in Dublin, Ireland, during my sabbatical several years ago. This recipe is the result of experimentation to maximize nutrition through the sourdough process and inclusion of whole wheat flour, while still maintaining the flavor and texture that my discriminating kids loved. This is a simple, traditional sourdough bread that you can feel good about serving your family.

If you are not using a scale, just skip over those portions of the recipe that describe how to measure ingredients in this way. Likewise, if you're not using a stand mixer, skip to the modification at the bottom of the recipe for instructions on how to mix by hand. You may notice the cup/gram equivalents vary from recipe to recipe in this book; for best results, use the amount indicated.

> 574 grams (2⅓ cups) water (about 75°F)
> 188 grams (1 cup) mature sourdough mother culture
>   (see page 128)
> 626 grams (4⅓ cups) bread flour
> 208 grams (1¼ cups) whole wheat or rye flour
> 20 grams (1 tablespoon) sea salt
> 188 grams (1 cup) sprouted grains, optional
> Rice flour, for dusting

Combine the water, sourdough mother, bread flour, and whole wheat flour in the bowl of a stand mixer fitted with the dough hook. Mix on speed 1 for 2 minutes, or until all the ingredients are thoroughly combined. Remove the dough hook, clean it, and set it aside. Cover the bowl of the stand mixer by placing a plate on top that fits snugly. Allow the dough to rest for 30 to 60 minutes.

Remove the plate from the bowl, add the salt, reattach the dough hook, and mix the dough on speed 2 for 3 minutes. If you're using the optional sprouted grains, add them now and mix for an additional 30 seconds to fully incorporate. You should see a change in the dough when it is ready: It should be tighter and smoother, and it should cling to the hook as a mass while it slaps against the side of the bowl.

Transfer the dough to a greased bowl, cover with a plate, and set aside to bulk-ferment for 2½ hours. Twice during the bulk fermentation stage, at the 50-minute mark and again at the 100-minute mark, give the dough a series of folds to further develop the gluten. To fold the dough, remove the plate and set aside, then dip one hand in a bowl of water to minimize sticking. Reach down inside the bowl along one side, grab the dough, and pull up to stretch. Stretch until you feel the gluten tighten, and stop just before the dough tears (see Figure 1). Complete the fold by laying the outstretched dough across the top of the dough. Turn the bowl 90 degrees and repeat. Continue until you have done this on all four sides. If the dough is sticking to the side of the bowl, it may be helpful to use a moistened scraper to dislodge the dough from the side before folding. Replace the plate and wait another 50 minutes, then repeat the folding.

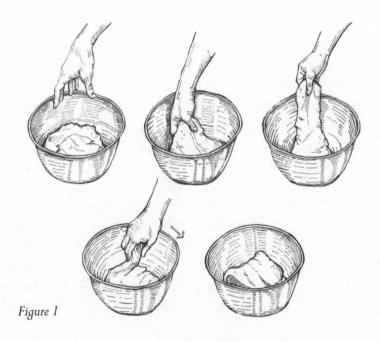

Figure 1

At the end of the bulk fermentation stage, lightly dust a work surface with flour, and leave a little pile of the flour nearby to work with. Divide the dough in half (or for buns, see the notes below) and place one half on the work surface. Place your hands on the far side of the dough, with your palms facing you and the fingertips of each hand touching one another. With the outside of your hands in contact with the work surface throughout the entire motion, slowly bring your hands toward you a few inches while gently pulling the mass of dough in the process (see Figure 2). The dough on the bottom will stick to the work surface and create a skin that stretches over the dough as you drag the mass over itself. If the dough slides instead of stretching, there is too much flour and you need to moisten the surface with a little water. If the dough is sticking to your hands, dip your palms in the pile of flour. Using a dough scraper, pick up the mass of dough and turn it 90 degrees, put it back down on the work surface, and again pull it over itself to tighten.

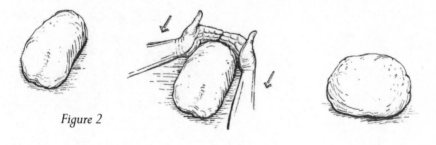

Figure 2

Now that you have done this in both directions, you should have created a fairly even ball with a smooth, slightly tight "skin" enveloping it. If not, repeat the steps one or two more times. Use the scraper to pick up the ball and place it out of the way on a lightly floured area of the work surface. Repeat with the other half of the dough and place it a few inches from the first one. Let the dough balls rest for 30 minutes so that the gluten relaxes for the next step and the surface dehydrates slightly to prevent it from sticking to the proofing basket later.

Use a sieve to lightly dust the insides of the proofing baskets with rice flour. If you do not have a proofing basket, you can line a bowl with a towel that has been well dusted with rice flour. Using your dough scraper, swiftly scoop up one of the balls of dough and place it upside down in the middle of your work surface. Brush off any excess flour. Imagine the dough as the face of a clock with 12 o'clock on the far side from you. Gently grab the far edge of the dough at 12 o'clock and bring the edge to the middle. Do the same at all of the even-numbered hours, 2, 4, 6, 8, and 10 (see Figure 3). This will allow you to easily and evenly tighten the dough and further shape the round. Turn the dough over so that the seam is on the bottom and use the same motions used during the pre-shaping stage to achieve a round shape with a tight surface. Invert and place in the proofing basket, seam side up. Repeat with the second ball of dough.

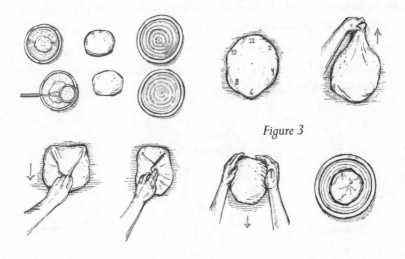

Figure 3

Cover and let sit in a warm place for 3 hours. While you are waiting for your bread to rise, cut a circle of parchment paper to fit inside the lid of a 5-quart Dutch oven (if you're using a pizza stone, the parchment is not necessary). An hour before you bake, place an oven rack in the center of the oven and carefully place your Dutch oven, upside down (with the lid on the bottom), on the rack. Preheat the oven to 500°F. (You will be baking with the Dutch oven inverted because it is easier and safer to transfer the dough to the shallower lid than to the deep pot itself.)

At the end of the 3 hours, place one of the baskets of dough, covered, in the refrigerator to slow the fermentation while the first loaf bakes. Use a sieve to lightly flour the exposed surface of the other dough. This exposed surface will be the bottom of your bread, and flouring it lightly will prevent it from sticking to your parchment. Place the parchment circle on top of the basket, followed by a cutting board or other sturdy, flat object. Pick up the basket, parchment, and cutting board as one unit and, with one hand underneath and one hand on top, quickly flip the entire stack upside down, placing everything back on the counter.

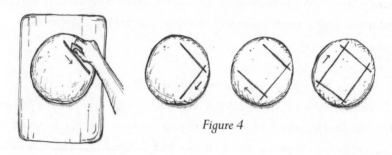

Figure 4

Remove the basket and gently reposition your dough so that it sits in the center of the parchment. Using a lame or serrated knife, swiftly score the top of the dough. One simple and common pattern is to score it four times in a hashtag pattern, with each cut about ½ inch deep (see Figure 4). Use heavy-duty oven mitts to open the door of your oven and pull out the Dutch oven. Remove the base and place it to the side. Position the cutting board, parchment paper, and dough over the Dutch oven lid. Hold the edge of the parchment with one hand and quickly pull the cutting board away with the other hand so that both the dough and the parchment drop, landing in the center of the lid (see Figure 5). Replace the base of the Dutch oven upside down on top of the lid and return the whole thing to the oven. Close the door and immediately reduce the oven temperature to 450°F.

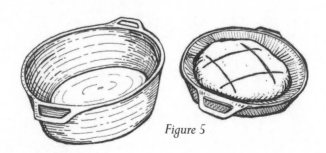

Figure 5

Bake for 20 minutes, then remove the base of the Dutch oven covering the bread. Continue to bake without a cover for another 20 to 25 minutes so that a crust forms and the bread browns. Remove the bread from the oven and place it on a rack to cool.

Place the entire Dutch oven back inside the oven and raise the heat back to 500°F. When preheated, remove the other dough from the refrigerator and repeat the transferring, scoring, and baking steps above.

Notes:

1. If you do not have a stand mixer, make the following adjustments:

Combine the water and sourdough mother in a large bowl and stir to evenly distribute. In a separate bowl, combine the flours and stir to evenly distribute. Add the dry ingredients to the wet ingredients, stir with a Danish dough whisk or wooden spoon until it becomes too difficult, then dump the contents out onto a clean work surface. Knead for several minutes by hand until all the ingredients are evenly distributed and the dough begins to come together. Place the dough in a clean bowl and cover with a plate for 30 to 60 minutes.

Add the salt and knead until the salt is evenly distributed and the dough is smooth and elastic.

Bulk-ferment for 2½ hours, but instead of folding the dough twice, at 50-minute intervals, fold the dough four times, at 30-minute intervals.

2. To make buns, divide the dough into 12 equal portions instead of 2, skip the final shaping step (pre-shaping into a round is enough), and bake on a pizza stone or baking sheet at 450°F for 15 to 20 minutes.

SOURDOUGH PRETZELS

Who doesn't love a warm soft pretzel straight out of the oven? Unfortunately, it is almost impossible to find a genuine sourdough pretzel, and many soft pretzels contain dozens of unhealthy ingredients. The good news is that they are easy to make at home, allowing you to control the ingredients and the process. Since these pretzels go through the sourdough process, they have all the same benefits as a rustic loaf of sourdough bread. Make these as a special treat that your family will love and you can feel good about.

Pretzels are dipped in a lye solution before baking to give them the brown, leathery crust we all love. However, working with lye can be dangerous, especially when cooking with your kids in the kitchen. Briefly boiling the pretzels in baking soda is a safer and more accessible alternative for our kitchens and is the process described below. If you want to learn more about using lye, visit eatlikeahuman.com.

- 800 grams (5 cups) bread flour
- 390 grams (1⅔ cups) water (about 75°F)
- 230 grams (1⅓ cups) mature sourdough mother culture (see page 128)
- 20 grams (1 tablespoon) sea salt
- 60 grams (⅓ cup) Fermented Butter (page 189) or store-bought unsalted butter, room temperature
- ½ cup baking soda
- Pretzel or kosher salt, for sprinkling

Combine the flour, water, sourdough mother, salt, and butter in the bowl of a stand mixer fitted with the dough hook. Mix on speed 1 for 3 minutes, then increase to speed 2 and mix for 6 minutes. If mixing by hand, combine all the ingredients and knead to create a smooth, elastic dough, about 10 minutes.

Transfer the dough to a greased bowl, cover with a plate, and set aside to bulk-ferment for 3½ hours. Once during the bulk fermentation, at the 1-hour mark, give the dough a series of folds. To fold the dough, remove the plate and set aside, then dip one hand in a bowl of water to minimize sticking. Reach down inside the bowl along one side, grab the dough, and pull up to stretch. Stretch until you feel the gluten tighten, and stop just before the dough tears (see Figure 1 on page 136). Complete the fold by laying the outstretched dough across the top of the dough. Turn the bowl 90 degrees and repeat. Continue until you have done this on all four sides. If the dough is sticking to the side of the bowl, it may be helpful to use a moistened scraper to dislodge the dough from the side before folding. Replace the plate.

At the end of the bulk fermentation, lightly dust a work surface with flour. Divide the dough into 10 equal portions. Pre-shape by rolling each piece of dough into a rope that measures 10 to 12 inches long, with tapered ends. Cover the dough ropes with a towel and rest for 20 minutes.

Shape by using slightly moistened hands to roll the dough again and increase the length of each rope to 16 inches. Take the two ends and cross them twice, then bring each down to meet the base to create a traditional pretzel shape. If the ends do not stick to the base, add a sprinkle of water to secure. Arrange the pretzels in a large container so that they're not touching, cover, and refrigerate overnight to slow the fermentation and firm up the dough to make handling easier.

The next day, preheat the oven to 350°F. Lightly grease a rimmed baking sheet. To prepare the alkaline bath, combine the baking soda with 2 quarts of water in a medium pot and bring to a boil over medium-high heat.

Remove the pretzels from the fridge and boil them, one at a time, in the alkaline bath for 15 to 20 seconds. Remove with a slotted spoon and drain, then place on the prepared baking sheet. Sprinkle with pretzel salt and bake for 20 to 25 minutes, until browned and leathery on the outside while soft and chewy on the inside.

SOURDOUGH PASTA

SERVES 4 TO 6

Pasta that comes out of a box is nothing more than boiled flour and has no place in our house. However, the kids love pasta, which prompted me to develop this recipe that solves two problems at the same time: The sourdough fermentation detoxifies and predigests the flour, and adding egg yolks skyrockets the nutritional value. For a quick midweek meal that can go directly from the freezer to boiling water, double or triple the recipe and freeze some after rolling and cutting out the pasta.

> 650 grams (5 cups) mature sourdough mother culture
> (see page 128)
> 650 grams (4½ cups) pasta flour (or flour of choice)
> 12 large egg yolks
> 20 grams (1 tablespoon) sea salt

Mix all the ingredients together in a large bowl with a Danish dough whisk or wooden spoon. Turn out the dough onto the counter and knead by hand until all the ingredients are incorporated and the dough is smooth. Wrap the dough in plastic wrap, or place it in a container large enough to allow for the dough to double in size during fermentation, and cover. Refrigerate for 6 to 12 hours to ferment.

Using a rolling pin or a pasta machine, roll out the pasta to a thickness of approximately ¹⁄₁₆ inch. Run through a pasta machine or cut by hand into the desired shape. Add a small amount of flour to keep the dough from sticking if needed.

Cook the pasta in boiling salted water immediately, or store in an airtight container in the fridge for a few days or in the freezer for several months.

SOURDOUGH PIZZA CRUST

MAKES 6 PIZZA CRUSTS

Christina and I built a wood-fired oven in our backyard more than 10 years ago. We were so excited to bake sourdough bread and make wood-fired pizzas entirely from scratch! However, for the first few years the kids didn't share our excitement. From charred bottoms to poorly made cheese, the kids suffered through years of subpar pizzas while we refused to order takeout. It wasn't until we learned from Chef John Nocita at the Italian Culinary Institute how to properly prepare and maintain the fire and cook the pizzas that we began to achieve success. Now, our pizzas are not only more beautiful and delicious than anything we could buy but incredibly healthy, too. Here is our go-to crust recipe, which I created by translating the Italian Culinary Institute pizza dough recipe into a sourdough one.

Our favorite way to use these crusts is to stretch or roll the dough into 12-inch-diameter rounds. Then we top them with a drizzle of extra virgin olive oil followed by minced garlic, salt, Mozzarella (page 192), Ricotta (page 203), and Fermented Roasted Red Peppers (page 54), then bake them in our wood-fired oven or on a pizza stone in our kitchen oven at 550°F for 10 to 15 minutes, until the cheese is melted and the crust is golden brown. Finish with arugula and balsamic vinegar as soon as they come out of the oven.

> 1,000 grams (7 cups) bread flour
> 508 grams (2¼ cups) water (about 75°F)
> 200 grams (1 cup) mature sourdough mother culture
>   (see page 128)
> 100 grams (⅓ cup plus 1 tablespoon) heavy cream
> 80 grams (⅓ cup plus 1 tablespoon) beer
> 30 grams (1½ tablespoons) sea salt
> 8 grams (1½ teaspoons) sugar

Combine all the ingredients in the bowl of a stand mixer fitted with the dough hook and mix on speed 1 for 2 minutes, then increase to speed 2 for 5 minutes. Remove the dough hook and place a large plate over the top of the bowl. Set the bowl aside to bulk-ferment for 2½ hours, giving it a series of folds every 30 minutes. To fold the dough, remove the plate and set aside, then dip one hand in a bowl of water to minimize sticking. Reach down inside the bowl along one side, grab the dough, and pull up to stretch. Stretch until you feel the gluten tighten, and stop just before the dough tears (see Figure 1 on page 136). Complete the fold by laying the outstretched dough across the top of the dough. Turn the bowl 90 degrees and repeat. Continue until you have done this on all four sides. If the dough is sticking to the side of the bowl, it may be helpful to use a moistened scraper to dislodge the dough from the side before folding. Replace the plate and wait another 30 minutes, then repeat the folding.

If you are not using a stand mixer, combine all the ingredients in a large bowl and mix with a Danish dough whisk or wooden spoon. Turn out the dough onto the counter and knead by hand to create a smooth, elastic dough, about 10 minutes, then follow the bulk fermenting and folding stage instructions above.

Divide the dough into six equal portions, shape into tight balls, and place in six individual bowls or other small containers. Cover with plastic wrap or lids and allow to rest at room temperature for 1½ hours.

Place the dough in the refrigerator overnight or for up to 2 days. Remove from the refrigerator 3 to 5 hours before using. (At this point, the dough can be wrapped tightly and frozen for several months. Make sure to thoroughly defrost and allow it to come to room temperature before using.)

SOURDOUGH CROUTONS

MAKES ABOUT 2 CUPS

Our Rise customers love these croutons! They're excellent on top of salads and soups, as a base for stuffing, or for a snack you can't put down. Olive oil and rosemary pair well for croutons and stuffing, and butter and Old Bay make an excellent complement to seafood chowder and crab dip.

    4 slices stale sourdough bread
    2 tablespoons extra virgin olive oil or melted butter
    Sea salt
    Dried rosemary, Old Bay, or other seasonings of choice (optional)

Preheat the oven to 250°F.

Cut the bread into cubes, toss with the olive oil or melted butter, and season with salt and your choice of seasonings, if desired. Spread out in a single layer on a rimmed baking sheet. Bake, tossing occasionally, until dry throughout and lightly browned, about 40 minutes. These can be used right away or stored in an airtight container at room temperature for several weeks.

GRANNY BREAD

MAKES 1 LOAF

My maternal grandmother, "Granny," would host dinner on Sunday nights. These were special events and cause for the entire family to dress up. She would serve appetizers of Wheat Thins and port wine cheddar cheese, mix cocktails for the adults, and make Jell-O filled with celery and walnuts. The highlight of the dinner, however, was the special bread that Granny served directly from the oven, tightly wrapped in aluminum foil. My sister, Heather, and I would fight over the butter-, garlic-, and spice-drenched slices in the middle. This bread has now become a staple for special occasions in my own home and my kids ask for it by name: Granny bread.

> 1 loaf Airfield Sourdough Bread (page 135) or other genuine
>   sourdough bread
> 1 cup Fermented Butter (page 189) or store-bought salted butter,
>   room temperature
> 2 teaspoons dried parsley, plus extra for garnish
> ½ teaspoon dried oregano
> ½ teaspoon dried dill
> 2 garlic cloves, minced
> 2 tablespoons grated Parmesan cheese

Preheat the oven to 400°F.

Cut the bread into 1-inch-thick slices. In a medium bowl, make a compound butter by blending together the butter, parsley, oregano, dill, and garlic. Spread the butter on each slice and reassemble the loaf. Wrap aluminum foil around the bottom, sides, and ends of the loaf, leaving the top open. Spread any remaining butter mixture on top and sprinkle with the Parmesan cheese and additional parsley. Warm in the oven for 15 minutes, or until all of the butter is melted and the top is browned.

Chapter 5

MAIZE

OR, THE CORN CONUNDRUM

We were late. The confused cab driver had driven 15 minutes in the wrong direction from our Airbnb before we realized the error, and it took another 10 minutes to convince him that we were heading the wrong way. Damn! We had been doing so well! In fact, Christina and I both felt like rock stars after having managed to get our entire family up, showered, fed, and out the door on time despite the previous 24 hours of mayhem. The day before Christmas Eve, one of the busiest travel holidays of the year, we had rushed home from work, grabbed the kids, loaded the truck, driven to the Philadelphia airport, and barely made it to the boarding gate on time. It was after 1 a.m. by the time we landed in Mexico City, collected our bags, found an Uber driver, and crashed blissfully into bed at our Airbnb. To successfully drag our jet-lagged family of five up and out of the house for an early morning class on traditional tortilla production—for which not all members of the Schindler clan equally shared my excitement— was a feat of heroic proportions.

Finally, after Christina and I teamed up with Google Maps and my broken Spanish to direct the driver, we arrived at Cal y Maíz, where founder Rigel Sotelo was waiting. He guided us around the back of the shop, past two women who were busy making tortillas, and upstairs to a platform loft he had set up as a classroom. At the last turn on the steps, we passed a shelf displaying a vivid array of different maize varieties—and suddenly I was catapulted back to being about seven years old, standing at Sickles

Farm in Little Silver, New Jersey. My mother, sister, and I were there to buy Halloween pumpkins, but I was captivated by that colorful, hard-shelled corn that Americans typically bundle up and hang on their front doors as an autumn decoration. "You don't want to eat *that*," one of the men working the register had said to me. "That's Indian corn. It's poisonous." That offhand, completely erroneous comment skewed my understanding of maize for decades.

You'll notice that I use the words *corn* and *maize* interchangeably, and they are, for all intents and purposes, the same. But the term *maize* is historically and scientifically more accurate. All corn as we know it today descends from New World maize (more on this later), and the word is derived from the Taino *mahiz* and Spanish *maíz*. It's also the scientific name: *Zea mays*. The word *corn* derives from an Old English word that means grain, and it may take on various meanings depending on geography; in Scotland and Ireland, oats are called corn, while in England, wheat is called corn. Maize, then, is a more precise term for what most Americans call corn, and also the more common word globally. But the malleability of the name also reflects my confusion surrounding this common food that began back at Sickles Farm, a lack of knowledge that eventually led me and my family to Mexico to learn more about maize and an ancient process called nixtamalization.

Nixtamalization: It's a lot of word to get your mouth around, but it's one you're going to want to know as you expand your knowledge of ancient food technologies and work to understand their importance in our contemporary diets. Because maize — corn — pervades your diet, whether you're conscious of it or not. It's in everything from salad dressing to cereal, mostly in the form of high-fructose corn syrup (HFCS). According to Tufts University's Friedman School of Nutrition Science and Policy, the average American consumes 160 pounds of corn annually, about 60 pounds of it in the form of high-fructose corn syrup. "Thanks mostly to the booming popularity of HFCS," the institution notes, "40 percent of all packaged, processed food sold in American supermarkets contains corn." How that affects our health — contributing to obesity, heart disease, and diabetes, among other illnesses — is an ongoing conversation in our culture, and if you're reading this book, chances are you are already well versed in the monster that maize has become in our diets. But how maize itself is processed can mean the difference between a healthy, nutritious food and one that can make you deathly ill.

If you think I'm exaggerating, consider the early 1900s in the southern United States, where steadily and inexorably, millions of people started getting sick. They developed terrible, disfiguring skin rashes when exposed to the sun. Their tongues grew swollen, their mouths bled, they suffered delusions and even dementia. Between 1907 and 1940, according to the National Institutes of Health (NIH), about three million Americans contracted the mysterious illness, and some 100,000 died. And this wasn't new. The same illness had first been described in Spain in 1735 by physician Don Gaspar Casal; it was mistaken for leprosy. Then it turned up in Italy in 1771, where it got its name—pellagra—which means rough or sour skin. It even made an appearance at the end of the potato famine in Ireland. The NIH notes that records in the US are sketchy, but by 1912, "the state of South Carolina alone reported 30,000 cases and a mortality rate of 40 percent." By way of comparison, by January 2021, the mortality rate in South Carolina from Covid-19 was just under 2 percent.

This sickness wasn't from a virus, and it baffled disease experts for generations. Since it affected impoverished areas more than others, it was thought to be an infectious "disease of filth." Not until 1917 did Dr. Joseph Goldberger finally prove that it was not infectious or viral but rather dietary, when he conducted experiments that involved participants eating corn-based diets versus diets based on fresh vegetables, meat, and milk. Those eating the corn-based diets exhibited pellagra symptoms within weeks; the others stayed healthy. Still, convincing other medical and health professionals was an uphill battle. Ultimately, he and his partner, Dr. George Wheeler, went so far as to inject themselves with the blood of infected victims to show that it wasn't a virus or germ that was causing the sickness. Even that was not enough, and Goldberger died in 1929 without having entirely solved the full mystery. Ten years later, scientists finally uncovered the commonality: a deficiency of niacin (vitamin B_3). As Goldberger had predicted, corn was the culprit. It explained why pellagra ended up even in Ireland, when maize, aka "Indian meal," was imported as famine relief food.

How on earth, you may be wondering, could a food as common as corn sicken and kill millions of people? And since it's clear that most people today aren't getting sick from pellagra (although it remains present in parts of the developing world, where people depend on maize as a staple food), why should we be concerned about corn in our diets today? The answers to these questions require us, again, to go back in time. And they serve as one of the starkest examples of how an ancient technology transformed a food that is difficult for humans to digest into something altogether more nutritious and bioavailable, and how we left that technology behind to our terrible detriment.

Archaeologists today believe that early peoples began domesticating maize more than 9,000 years ago in the Balsas Valley of Mexico, from a wild grass called teosinte. The genetic selections and modifications that have occurred over time have transformed wild teosinte into the maize we know today. Early forms of maize were small and had kernels that were individually encased in husks — they looked like shaggy clumps of fur, all clinging to a central stem — and they were laborious and time-consuming to clean. Changes to maize over time created a cob that is much larger and covered by one husk, drastically reducing harvesting and processing time. Today, maize comes in a variety of forms, from so-called Indian corn — the multicolored corn I saw that day long ago at Sickles Farm in New Jersey — to feed corn for animals, popcorn, and sweet corn that comes to us on cobs or in cans.

Anywhere maize has been introduced over millennia, it has come to dominate diets because it is filling, affordable, and easy to grow. The most widely produced crop in the world, grown in at least 164 countries, maize had a total production of more than 1 billion metric tons in 2019. It is the largest crop in the United States, with nearly 92 million acres of it planted in 2019, according to the USDA National Agricultural Statistics Service, ahead of soybeans by about 8 million acres. Nearly a third of those 92 million acres produced maize that went into our diets (another third was used for livestock feed grain, and the final third in ethanol). Maize is the basis of hundreds of foods, such as grits, breakfast cereal, polenta, and corn-meal, and it permeates processed foods in the form of high-fructose corn syrup and cornstarch.

Yet, maize presents a conundrum. It's one of the hardest foods for our bodies to digest. The main component of its cell walls is indigestible cellulose. And although it contains high levels of niacin, this important vitamin remains locked away and inaccessible to our bodies unless maize is processed in a specific way. Early Mesoamerican farmers unknowingly stumbled onto this when they began to process maize by simmering dried kernels in a solution of water and wood ash, then steeping the mixture overnight. This is the first step in the process of nixtamalization. The next day, they could more easily remove the kernels' hard outer coatings. Then they rinsed the grains; at this point, the product is called nixtamal or hominy. Nixtamal could be used as is, coarsely ground into hominy grits, or finely ground into a highly digestible, nutritious dough called masa. Today, masa is used in a number of traditional ways: pressed into tortillas, formed into tamales—which bear the name of the process itself—and even mixed into a delicious and nourishing drink known as atole. Combined with beans, nixtamalized maize provides a complete protein.

Over time, calcium hydroxide (commonly known as cal, pickling lime, hydrated lime, or slacked lime) and, on industrial levels, even sodium hydroxide (commonly known as lye) replaced wood ash (potassium hydroxide). But the process has remained the same and so has the result: The mixture of a base, like cal, with water creates an alkaline solution that chemically and physically transforms maize into its safest and most nourishing form possible for our digestive tracts. Through nixtamalization, these grains are detoxified. The process neutralizes antinutrients such as phytic acid, raises the calcium content by up to 400 percent, increases the protein quality by improving the amino acid balance and digestibility, and releases niacin from its bound form, which is unavailable to our bodies. Descendants of those early Mesoamerican farmers continue to use this process, and though maize is still a staple of their diet, they remain free of pellagra. When you skip nixtamalization, no matter how you cook corn, much of its nutrition stays locked up in the grain, which

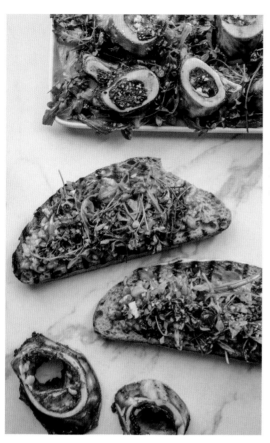

Wild Greens, Roasted Bone Marrow, and Sourdough (page 38)

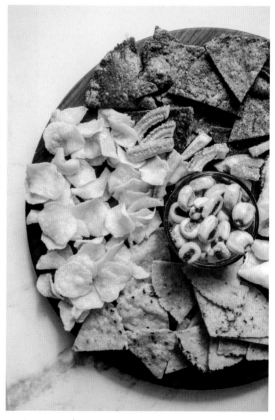

Lacto-Chips (page 56), Nix 'Nacks (page 163), Tortilla Chips (page 162), Back Fat Cracklins (page 95), Pork Rinds (page 93)

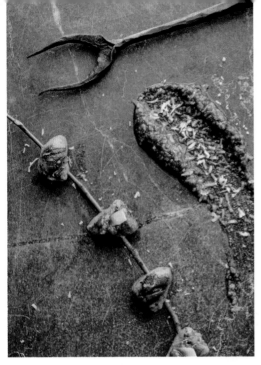

Grilled Chicken Hearts with
Wild Pesto (page 83)

Fried Chicken Wings (page 85),
Bola's Blue Cheese Dressing (page 87),
Fermented Carrot Sticks, and Celery

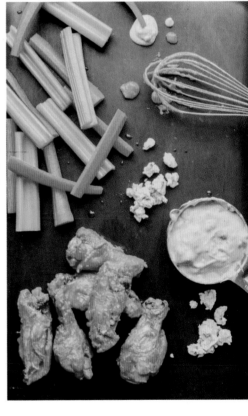

Chicken Caesar Salad with Crispy
Chicken Skins (page 90)

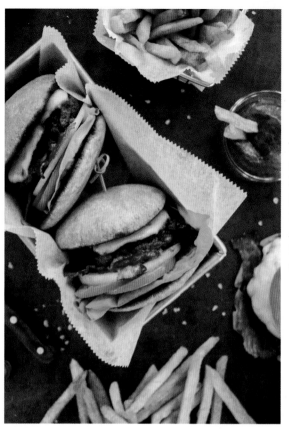

The Ultimate Nose-to-Tail Burger (page 99), Mozzarella (page 192), Modern Stone Age Kitchen Bacon (page 97), Fermented Ketchup (page 101), Lettuce, Tomato, and Onion on Airfield Sourdough Bread Buns (page 135) with Lacto-Fries (page 56) and Charcoal Mayonnaise (page 240)

Chocolate Overnight Oats and Citrus Overnight Oats (page 120)

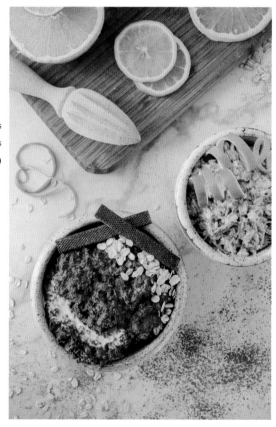

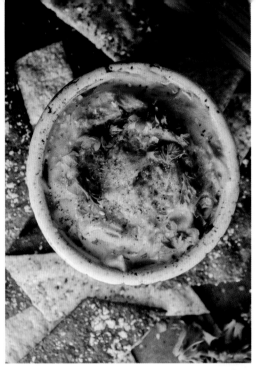

Avi's Traditional Hummus (page 123) with Butter Bite Crackers (page 133), and Charcoal Crackers (page 237)

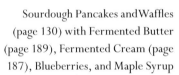

Sourdough Pancakes and Waffles (page 130) with Fermented Butter (page 189), Fermented Cream (page 187), Blueberries, and Maple Syrup

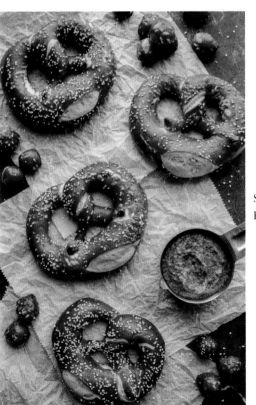

Sourdough Pretzels (page 141) with Fermented Mustard (page 103)

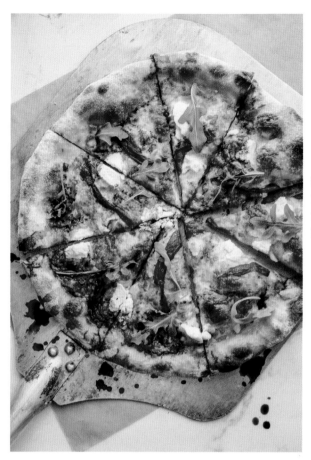

Sourdough Pizza Crust (page 144) with Mozzarella (page 192), Ricotta, and Fermented Roasted Red Peppers (page 54)

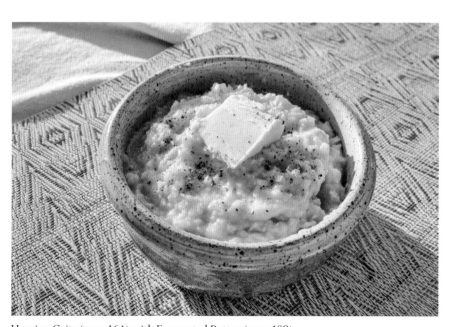

Hominy Grits (page 164) with Fermented Butter (page 189)

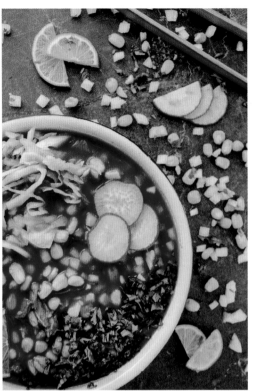

Pozole (page 165) with Amazing Sauerkraut (page 50)

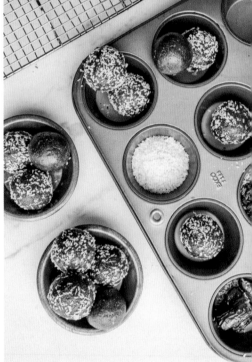

Cricket Power Balls (page 217)

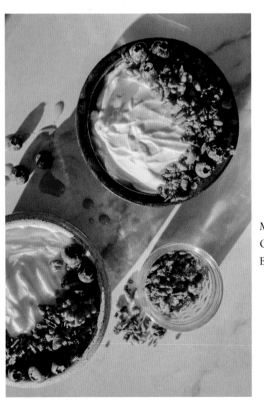

Mesophilic Yogurt (page 183), Cricket Granola (page 219), and Blueberries

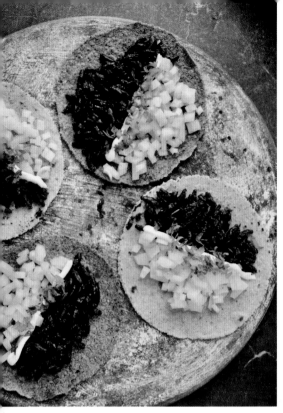

Tacos with Tortillas (page 160),
Chili-Lime Crickets (page 221),
Fermented Cream (page 187),
Raw Onion, and Cilantro

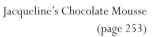

Jacqueline's Chocolate Mousse
(page 253)

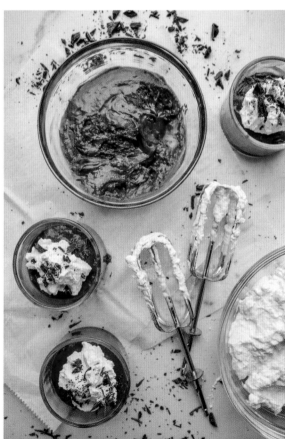

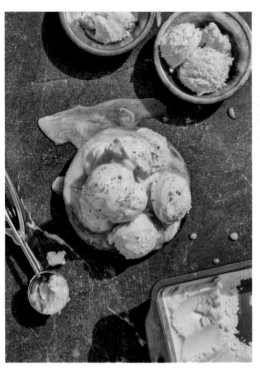

Honey Ice Cream (page 255) with
Fermented Honey (page 257) and
Bee Pollen

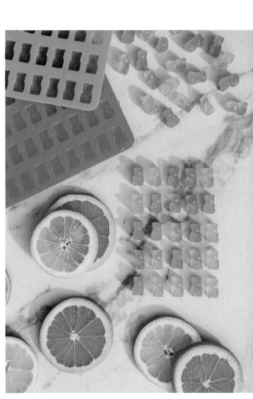

Healthy Gummies
(page 258)

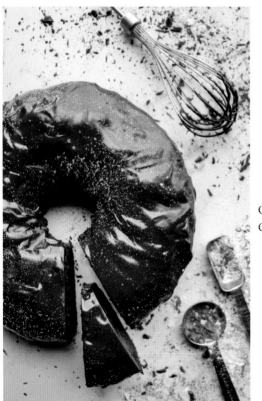

Chocolate Maple Sourdough
Cake with Ganache (page 260)

simply navigates our digestive tracts and gets expelled, taking its nutrition with it.

So, if Mesoamerican people's process made maize a safe and nutritious staple food for thousands of years, how did pellagra become so devastating in the United States? Even while people in Mesoamerica were processing maize in this way, their traditional techniques did not accompany the growth of global maize consumption. Instead, simple grinding and cooking processes were developed that kept important nutrients locked within the maize, passing unabsorbed through our bodies and leading to malnutrition and niacin deficiency. This became dangerous and common anywhere that maize—which is cheap, filling, and adaptable to growing in a variety of regions—dominated the diet to the exclusion of other food and essential nutrients. Anywhere in the world, including the southern United States, where corn became a foundation of diet but traditional nixtamalization techniques didn't travel with it, pellagra followed. Even today, people in developing countries who depend largely on maize still suffer from this—literally getting sick and dying from a niacin deficiency, even while eating large amounts of a food that contains plenty of niacin! Yet when we finally discovered the problem, we didn't return to nixtamalization as part of the process. Instead we began to artificially enrich maize-based foods with niacin. And this remains how we address the issue today, while continuing to seek innovations and genetic modifications of maize to solve the problem, rather than adopting a process proven over thousands of years.

The more I learned about nixtamalization's ability to transform corn into the most nutrient-dense, bioavailable food it could be, the more I wanted to know. For me, there's no substitute for learning directly from experts and using all of my senses to see, smell, hear, feel, and taste my way through a process. That's why I had packed up the family and dragged them down to Mexico, and why we found ourselves at Cal y Maíz, where Rigel began our education by explaining that while more than 64 different varieties of corn are under cultivation in Mexico, all of them—in fact *all* varieties of corn grown around the world—come from a single variety of teosinte. He postulated that early farmers began nixtamalizing maize thousands of years ago not because they had a clue about niacin deficiency, but because they noticed that water boils faster when you add ash to it — saving time and fuel. During the workshop, we learned how to shell the olote (cob) by hand and with an oloteras, a traditional device made from leftover cobs bound together in a circle, which looked less like a tool than artwork. We watched as one of Rigel's top tortilla makers demonstrated grinding maize on the metate, an ancient stone tool that she had grown up using with her mother every day to grind masa for her family. To show us how nixtamal is quickly turned into masa for commercial purposes, Rigel fired up the mechanized version of the metate, the molino — a machine that uses a 1.5-horsepower motor to rotate two grinding stones. We learned the finer points of tortilla making and cooking, and then we mingled traditional recipes — like tacos with quesillo (Oaxacan string cheese) and epazote, a Mexican herb related to lamb's quarters — with contemporary gourmet versions that included fillings such as huitlacoche (a fungus that grows on corn and is considered a delicacy in Mexico), roasted bone marrow, and ant eggs.

Cal y Maíz provided a terrific opportunity for hands-on experience producing delicious and healthy tortillas on a modern, commercial scale. But I also wanted to see what this process looked like when used by a traditional family as part of their daily lives and diets. So, a few days later, we traveled high into the mountains of southwestern Mexico, where we spent a day with Juana, Emiliano, and their family, who lived in San Antonio de la Cal in a spotlessly clean, dirt-floored home made of recycled wood and corrugated tin. (Their town is so named because it's literally built on a mountain of cal, which they harvest directly from the ground.) They showed us how they process their maize, starting with a palmful of cal that Emiliano pulled from a bag filled with white, chalk-like chunks of powdery rock. This was the perfect amount to nixtamalize 6 kilos of maize kernels, which is how much they process every other day to provide their family of five enough tortillas to last two days. He put the cal in a small bowl of water, which immediately began to bubble. Once the chemical reaction subsided, Juana added the mixture to a metal bucket containing maize kernels and additional water, then moved the bucket to the outdoor kitchen, where she balanced it atop a circle of rocks, under which burned a wood-fueled fire. After letting it boil for about an hour, Juana removed the bucket and set it aside, where it would steep till the next day. So that we could see the whole process, she moved to a second bucket containing maize that had already steeped overnight. Rubbing the kernels between her hands, she removed the skins and washed the nixtamal repeatedly until the water was clear.

Then, Emiliano handed me the bucket of nixtamal and motioned me toward a gate; we had only a short window of time to grind this nixtamal, now that it had been washed. We headed for the molino, the community's beating heart, where everyone gathers to transform their nixtamal into masa. Several women from the village were already there, their musical voices in constant and lively conversation, offsetting the clattering of the machine. They worked in fluid teams of three: one to monitor the distance between the molino's grinding stones, which dictates the consistency of the final masa; one to feed the kernels from the hopper and regulate the thin stream of water that helps hydrate the masa and lubricate the machine; and a third to keep the grinding stones clear and scrape the drum clean. As people came and went and the molino rumbled nonstop, it was clear that like a local pub in a small town, this central processing facility was the place where everyone gathered at one point or another to talk, make plans, tell stories, and connect with one another. One by one women, children, and families dropped off their nixtamal to be ground, checked in with their neighbors and friends, and then headed home with their transformed food, now a smooth, moist dough that reminded me of moldable clay. They wrapped their masa in beautifully woven blankets and placed it in baskets for transport. Emiliano explained that each family's masa is slightly different, determined by how much cal they use and how long they cook the cal and maize. These two variables affect nuances of the final flavor, texture, and color of the tortillas and represent an excellent way to maintain family identity while also engaging in a communal activity like the molino.

Our day with Emiliano and Juana ended with — what else — beautifully prepared food. On a huge ceramic comal — a round, flat griddle — over an open fire, Juana dry-roasted a few peppers and garlic, which she expertly crushed into a salsa in a ceramic bowl made for the job. Her daughter used a tortilla press to create tlayudas, extra-large tortillas typical of this region. We cooked, shared stories, and traded experiences and cultures. Through a simple tortilla, we learned about and connected with a generous family, an entire village, and a process that is thousands of years old and can still be used to improve our contemporary diets.

Today, since baked goods are fortified with niacin, we can safely eat as many corn-based products as we want without developing pellagra—although, if you eat enough processed foods that contain high-fructose corn syrup, you'll have other health problems to deal with. But knowing the clear benefits of nixtamalization, it makes enormous sense to use nixtamalized maize whenever and wherever you can to reap the maximum nutrition from this ubiquitous and ancient grain. As an educated consumer, you can choose products that use only corn that has been nixtamalized; Bob's Red Mill masa harina, for instance, clearly states on the label that it's made from nixtamalized corn. And to connect more directly with our dietary past and empower your own health, you can easily nixtamalize your own maize at home and use it for everything from tortillas and pozole to corn nuts and chips.

TIPS AND RECIPES

HOW TO SHOP FOR THE BEST TORTILLAS

Ideally, you will make your own tortillas from maize you have nixtamalized and turned into amazing masa. But if that's not an option, here are some tips for how to buy the next best thing:

- Purchase tortillas from a store. Some stores (especially Mexican or Hispanic grocery stores) offer fresh or frozen tortillas. Read the label. If the only ingredients are maize, an alkaline ingredient (cal, hydrated lime, or calcium hydroxide), and water, they are worth purchasing.

- Purchase tortillas from a local tortilleria that has a molino on site to ensure they are nixtamalizing their own maize.
- Make your own tortillas from commercially available masa flour, or dried nixtamalized maize. The ingredients list should have only maize and an alkaline ingredient (cal, hydrated lime, or calcium hydroxide). The downside to this option is that most masa flour has been degerminated, so the most nutrient-rich part of the maize is missing. It's akin to the difference between whole wheat flour and white flour.

BAKING WITH MASA

For a special treat, add leftover masa to your flour the next time you bake bread. It will give the bread a unique taste and texture and increase its nutritional value. Because masa is moist, you can add up to 20 percent of the total weight of the flour and not throw off the dough's flour/water ratio. In other words, you can safely add 20 grams of masa to 100 grams of flour with no additional adjustments. See the Masa Sourdough Bread recipe on page 167.

PLASTIC AND TORTILLAS?

We all want to remove plastic from our lives. But there are a few situations in the kitchen when plastic makes it much easier to get a superior final product, and making tortillas is one of them. Masa dough is slightly sticky, and whether you are using a tortilla press or a rolling pin, you need to put something between each side of the dough to allow it to release. Believe it or not, the cheapest, thinnest plastic (think grocery store bags) works best. Flatten the bag, place it in the press, and trace the circular edge of the press with a marker. Cut what you've traced with a pair of scissors; you will be left with two circles (both sides of the bag). If you're not using a press, you can still use this technique to roll out your tortillas with a rolling pin. If you really don't want to use plastic, you can substitute waxed paper or parchment.

NIXTAMAL/HOMINY

The physical and chemical changes that take place when maize is heated in an alkaline solution are nothing short of magical. This process transforms maize from a bland, nutritionally inaccessible, boring grass seed into a nourishing, delicious, aromatic, and prehistoric and historic staple in many parts of the Americas. Known by several different names, such as nixtamal and hominy, the product of this ancestral technology is the first step toward producing foods such as Tortillas (page 160), Hominy Grits (page 164), and Pozole (page 165). Dried maize and cal can be found online at masienda.com.

10 cups (2,366 grams) water
4 cups (800 grams) dried maize (corn) kernels
1½ tablespoons (12 grams, or 1.5% of the weight of the corn)
    cal or pickling lime

Combine the water, maize, and cal or pickling lime in a large pot. Stir to combine and bring to a simmer over medium-high heat. Reduce the heat and simmer for about 30 minutes. There are two tests to alert you when it is ready. First, take a kernel and rub it between your fingers. The skin should slip off. Next, place the kernel in your mouth and bite gently. It should have the texture of al dente pasta.

When ready, turn off the heat, cover, and let steep overnight (about 12 hours). After steeping, drain the corn in a colander and rub it between your hands to break up some of the dissolved skin; now the maize is properly called nixtamal. Rinse the nixtamal in water. The skins will drain with the water through the holes in the colander. Repeat rubbing the kernels with your hands and rinsing to remove more skins. If you are making hominy for recipes such as Pozole, Hominy Grits, and Nix 'Nacks, continue to rinse until all of the skins are completely removed. If you are going to grind into masa, repeat rubbing and rinsing only until about half of the skins are removed. The remaining gelatinized skins help the final masa dough stick together and also contribute to the unique flavor of traditional tortillas.

Nixtamal should be ground into masa the same day it is rinsed, preferably within a few hours, then wrapped tightly to keep it from drying out and used within 24 hours. Hominy (nixtamal with all the skins removed) can be stored, covered, in the refrigerator for up to 1 week or in the freezer for several months.

TORTILLAS

MAKES ABOUT 24

Ideally, nixtamal is ground into masa by hand on a stone metate or mechanically on an electric molino. Making masa with stone grinds the nixtamal and also "smears" it into a smooth paste. However, with a few modifications, you can make excellent masa with the equipment you already have in your kitchen. Your food processor will break down the nixtamalized kernels into a smooth dough, but it does so by cutting instead of grinding and smearing—not ideal, but OK. Also, the motors in food processors cannot handle thick dough, so you may need to add a little extra water to allow it to work long enough to break it down fine. If that is the case, the resulting dough will be a little too wet for tortillas; you can reduce the hydration/stickiness by spreading it out and letting it dry a bit or by adding a little commercial masa flour.

> 4 cups nixtamal
> Water, as needed

Transfer a small amount of the nixtamal to a food processor. Do not overfill! The dough it creates is very thick, and too much will overwork the processor's motor. Process until it is a smooth dough. You may need to add small amounts of water, about a teaspoon at a time, to get everything to combine and grind properly. When it is smooth, remove the masa dough from the food processor and, if not too wet, wrap or place in a covered container to ensure it does not lose moisture. Continue with the remainder of the nixtamal until it has all been ground.

Preheat a griddle or skillet to high heat. You can use a tortilla press to create your tortillas; lining each side of the press with plastic makes it easier to remove them. If you don't have a press, take a small ball of the masa and flatten it between two pieces of plastic with your hands or with a rolling pin. Gently transfer the tortilla to the preheated griddle and cook for a few seconds on the first side, then flip the tortilla and cook for a few minutes on the second side. When ready, flip back to the original side to finish cooking. The tortilla should fill with air like a balloon. If it doesn't, don't worry—it will still be the most nutritious and delicious tortilla you've ever had! When it has finished cooking, remove it from the griddle and wrap it in a kitchen towel. Repeat with the remaining dough, carefully stacking the finished tortillas on top of one another in the towel.

Finished tortillas can be wrapped and stored in the refrigerator for up to 1 week or in the freezer for up to 3 months (they store best vacuum-sealed). To use, reheat both sides on a hot griddle.

TORTILLA CHIPS

MAKES ABOUT 60

By definition, tortilla chips are supposed to be made from nixtamalized maize, while corn chips are made from simply ground maize. So, from a nutrient bioavailability perspective, tortilla chips are a better choice. However, it is impossible to find any that haven't been fried in unhealthy oils, so the best option is to make them yourself from homemade or high-quality purchased tortillas.

Stale tortillas can easily be made into delicious tortilla chips that retain the nutritional advantages of the nixtamalization process. And when they are deep-fried in animal fat instead of industrial nut and seed oils, they become a much healthier alternative to anything you can find in the chips aisle in the grocery store.

2 quarts animal fat (such as lard or tallow)
10 stale tortillas
Sea salt

Melt enough animal fat in a deep fryer or large, heavy pot to completely submerge the chips, while not going any higher than halfway up the pot. Heat the fat to 300°F. Cut each tortilla into 6 pie-shaped wedges and deep-fry for 5 minutes, or until dry, crisp, and slightly browned. Drain and salt while still warm. Once cooled, they can be eaten right away or stored in an airtight container at room temperature for up to 1 week.

NIX 'NACKS

MAKES ABOUT 2 CUPS

The combination of nixtamalization and frying in animal fat makes this homemade version of corn nuts much healthier than anything you can buy at the store. By changing up the spice mixture you can create everything from Old Bay seasoning to salt-and-pepper versions.

> 2 quarts animal fat (such as lard or tallow)
> 2 cups fresh nixtamal, rinsed and drained
> Sea salt
> Old Bay, freshly ground black pepper, garlic salt, and/or other
> seasonings of choice (optional)

Melt enough fat in a deep fryer or large, heavy pot to completely submerge the kernels, while not going any higher than halfway up the pot. Heat the fat to 350°F.

Spread out the nixtamal on a rimmed baking sheet lined with paper towels. Pat the surface with additional paper towels. It is important to remove as much surface moisture as possible to reduce splattering in the hot fat. Let the kernels sit, exposed to the air, while the fat heats up in your fryer.

Deep-fry in batches until brown and crisp, about 6 minutes. When the kernels have taken on a rich brown color, remove them from the fat and spread them out on a wire rack, crumpled paper bag, or paper towels. Immediately season with salt and spices, if desired, while still warm. Allow to cool and enjoy. Nix 'nacks can be stored in a sealed container at room temperature for several weeks.

HOMINY GRITS

Grits, a staple in the south, were traditionally made from hominy, and *hominy* is actually just another word for nixtamal. However, things began to change after the Civil War, when, for a variety of reasons, ground corn replaced hominy grits, thereby not conveying all of nixtamalized maize's nutrition. Today, there is a great deal of confusion surrounding grits, hominy grits, hominy, polenta, mush, and cornmeal. It's difficult to make sense of the labels and much easier to simply make them yourself. Plus, it is a great way to use up the nixtamal that you didn't get a chance to grind into masa.

2 cups nixtamal

3 cups milk and/or water

2 tablespoons butter, plus more for serving

1 cup shredded cheddar cheese (optional)

Sea salt and freshly ground black pepper

Pulse the nixtamal in a food processor until there are no longer any whole kernels. The finer the grind, the creamier the grits; the coarser the grind, the toothier the bite.

Transfer the grits to a large skillet and cook over medium heat, stirring, until they begin to toast and you can smell them. Meanwhile, in a small saucepan, heat the milk and/or water to a simmer over low heat. Once the milk is hot and the grits aromatic, begin to add hot milk to the grits, ½ cup at a time, stirring constantly and making sure the milk is fully absorbed by the grits before adding the next round. Once all the milk has been added, turn off the heat and add the butter and optional cheese. Stir until melted, then season with salt and pepper to taste.

POZOLE

SERVES 8 TO 10

The first time I tried pozole, I fell in love with it. What's not to love? It is a warm, nourishing stew that is easy to make and uses nixtamalized maize. While traditionally made with pork, just about any meat, from wild game to chicken, will work in this recipe. Plus, it is a great way to use nixtamal/hominy without having to grind it into masa.

4 quarts water

3 pounds boneless meat (pork shoulder, pork belly, venison, beef, or chicken), cut into 2-inch pieces

1 bay leaf

½ teaspoon whole black peppercorns

1 tablespoon fresh oregano, preferably Mexican, plus more for garnish

1 onion, chopped, divided

6 garlic cloves, peeled

5 dried guajillo peppers, seeded

5 dried ancho peppers, seeded

8 cups nixtamal or store-bought hominy

3 tablespoons lard or butter

Sea salt

Optional garnishes: lime wedges, sliced radishes, fermented cabbage

Combine the water and cubed meat in a large stockpot and bring to a boil over medium-high heat. Skim the surface and reduce to a simmer. Add the bay leaf, peppercorns, oregano, half of the onion, and 4 of the garlic cloves. Continue simmering for 1 hour, or until the meat easily pulls apart.

While the broth is simmering, combine the seeded guajillo and ancho peppers, remaining onion, and remaining 2 garlic cloves in a medium heatproof bowl.

When the broth is finished, strain it through a colander into another pot or a large bowl, clean the stockpot, and return the broth to it. Ladle enough of the hot, strained broth into the bowl containing the peppers, onion, and garlic to cover. Set the bowl aside for 30 minutes to rehydrate the peppers. Shred the meat with your fingers or two forks and return the shredded meat, along with the onion and garlic, to the pot. Add the nixtamal or hominy to the pot. Return to a simmer over medium heat.

When the peppers have rehydrated, strain the peppers, onion, and garlic through a sieve into a bowl and place in a blender. Add 2 cups of the strained liquid to the blender and pour the remaining strained liquid into the pot. Puree the peppers, onion, garlic, and liquid until smooth. Heat the lard or butter in a sauté pan over medium-high heat and add the puree. Stir to incorporate the fat, then reduce to a simmer and continue to cook for 30 minutes. Add the mixture to the stockpot and stir to incorporate. Season with salt to taste.

Ladle the pozole into bowls and garnish as desired.

MASA SOURDOUGH BREAD

This recipe is based on my Airfield Sourdough Bread recipe (page 135). If you are not using a stand mixer, skip to the modification at the bottom of the Airfield Sourdough Bread recipe for instructions on how to mix by hand.

> 574 grams (2⅓ cups) water (approximately 75°F)
> 188 grams (1 cup) mature sourdough mother culture
>   (see page 128)
> 188 grams (¾ cup) fresh masa
> 626 grams (4⅓ cups) bread flour
> 208 grams (1¼ cups) whole wheat or rye flour
> 20 grams (1 tablespoon) sea salt
> Rice flour, for dusting

Combine the water, sourdough mother, fresh masa, bread flour, and whole wheat flour in the bowl of a stand mixer fitted with the dough hook. Mix on speed 1 for 2 minutes, or until the ingredients are thoroughly combined. Remove the dough hook, clean it, and set it aside. Cover the bowl of the stand mixer by placing a plate on top that fits snugly. Allow the dough to rest for 30 to 60 minutes.

Remove the plate from the bowl, add the salt, reattach the dough hook, and mix the dough on speed 2 for 3 minutes. You should see a change in the dough when it is ready; it should be tighter and smoother, and it should cling to the hook as a mass while it slaps against the side of the bowl. Transfer to a greased bowl, cover with a plate, and set aside to bulk-ferment for 2½ hours.

The rest of this recipe is the same as the Airfield Sourdough Bread, page 137. Follow the remainder of the steps there to complete the recipe.

Chapter 6

DAIRY

THE FOUNDATIONAL FOOD

For the past 16 years, I have been breaking the law.

This happens every time I drive from my home in Maryland to Pennsylvania, where I stop at the Wawa to get ice, roll my truck down the Amish farm's driveway, and collect my eight gallons of raw milk from the farmer before returning home. Maryland is one of many states in the US that ban the sale and use of raw milk for human consumption. So, to provide my family with what I feel is the most nutritious and safest milk, I have to do something illegal.

The raw milk debate in America continues to rage, as well it should. What used to be the norm in dairy-based communities for more than 10,000 years is not only obscure today but illegal in most of the country. Raw milk is fresh, full of nutrition, and chock-full of the natural bacteria required to kick-start and support a variety of fermentations that can transform it into a range of safe, nutrient-dense, and bioavailable foods. Yet, most people think that the only safe way to drink milk is to get it after it has been pasteurized—that is to say, stripped of anything living, which includes beneficial bacteria and enzymes. On the one hand, this seems logical, since none of us wants to consume dangerous bacteria. On the other, it flies in the face of what has been a healthy and reliable food source for almost 10,000 years.

So how have we gone so far astray from our ancestral relationship with milk and dairy? How is it that we question whether milk is a healthy part of our diets today? And, how can we relearn traditional techniques that make milk — and all of the wonderful foods we can create with it, from cheese and yogurt to butter and kefir — as safe and nutritious as possible?

To start to answer these questions, we have to start at the beginning: birth. For at least 200 million years — since our first mammalian ancestors evolved — we have consumed milk at birth and as infants. We think of this milk as the beneficial powerhouse that it is, fueling and supporting one of the most nutritionally critical periods of our lives. What we don't think about is that even as we drink it, this milk — teeming with beneficial bacteria — is in the process of fermenting. In our bodies, it encounters a variety of enzymes that change it chemically and physically. Lactase helps digest lactose, the sugar found in milk. Lipase helps break down the fat. And chymosin-like enzymes help thicken the milk so that it stays in our digestive system longer, giving our body more time to absorb its nutrition. Not to be overly graphic, but have you noticed how, when a baby spits up milk, it smells a lot like a zesty provolone cheese? That's because it basically is just that: cheese. As we digest our mother's milk, bacterial fermentation is transforming it into the safest, most nutritious food it can be. (Keep this in mind when we discuss cheesemaking a little further along.) As we grow older, our bodies lose some of those enzymes that make milk more easily digestible. Over 65 percent of the human population develops lactose intolerance after infancy, a situation that results in stomach pain, bloating, gas, and diarrhea. As with wheat gluten and bread, simply eliminating milk and dairy products from our diets is seen as a solution. But I would argue this is the wrong approach. Instead, we should approach milk and dairy products the same way we humans have approached every other food in our dietary past — not *if* we should eat them, but rather *how*.

There is no doubt that early hunter-gatherers, who used every part of the animal, consumed milk from mammary glands of the lactating animals they killed. We know that our ancestors had access to the milk of other animals at least 49,000 years ago; this is the date of art in Witwatersrand Cave in Johannesburg, South Africa, for which the natural pigment ochre was mixed with milk, likely obtained from a lactating bovid (a mammal from the cattle family). However, direct evidence of milk consumption from animals harvested by hunter-gatherers is difficult to identify in the archaeological record. Instead, we can turn to historic ethnographic studies as proxy evidence to help understand how our ancestors, who epitomized the nose-to-tail approach to their kills, may have operated. For instance, the Hare, also known as Kawchottine, living in northwestern Canada "are reported to relish moose mammary glands when the female is lactating in the summer," according to anthropologist Hiroko Hara. Likewise, the Chippewa savored the udders of "milk-giving does" so much that they consumed them on the spot when an animal was killed. Anthropologist Lorna Marshall documented how the !Kung bushmen of the Kalahari would give the udders from their kills to the elderly because they were soft. In the 1969 ethnography *Food and Emergency Food in the Circumpolar Area,* anthropologist Kerstin Eidlitz Kuoljok recorded how the Iglulik Inuit cooked ringed seal pup stomachs when they were full of milk after they nursed from their mothers and noted how the final product tasted like cheese. John J. Honigmann reported that the Kaska from northeastern British Columbia and southeastern Yukon drank moose milk. (I have had deer milk myself; the milk was delicious and full of fat. In fact, while cow's milk contains on average 4 percent fat, milk from deer is between 10 and 20 percent fat.)

While our hunter-gatherer ancestors likely found milk a rewarding, if unpredictable, byproduct of hunting, it didn't make much of an impact on their diets. Instead, the archaeological record suggests that we started regularly consuming milk from other animals between 8,000 and 10,000 years ago, when our ancestors first started domesticating milk-producing animals. We likely weren't drinking milk, but we were using it as the basis for an array of other dairy products, including yogurt, butter, kefir, and cheese. Similar to what happens inside an infant's stomach, lactobacillus fermentation (lacto-fermentation for short) occurs naturally when milk is not refrigerated but rather is left to sit out, and since we know that our early ancestors didn't have Sub-Zeros or Frigidaires, we can infer that they observed this. Lacto-fermentation happens when lactobacillus bacteria, so-called friendly bacteria, convert sugars in foods into lactic acid. In the case of dairy, these bacteria use lactase — the enzyme that many people lose the ability to produce over time—to break down the sugar lactose. The result is a different food: Fermentation reduces or eliminates lactose; increases beneficial bacteria and yeasts (what we call probiotics); boosts acidity, which fends off pathogens; predigests the milk, making it easier to metabolize; increases B vitamins; and improves its aroma, flavor, and texture.

Kefir provides a good example of the probiotics that can be present in a fermented dairy product. Though this will vary depending on how the kefir is made, in general, there are at least seven predominant bacteria species in kefir—among them *Lactobacillus acidophilus* and *Lactobacillus kefiri*— as well as two dozen species of yeast. From a more practical standpoint, lacto-fermentation also enabled our forebears to transform a perishable food into storable, nutrient-dense, bioavailable products that had pleasing yet distinct tastes, smells, and textures. These butters, cheeses, kefirs, and yogurts became important food resources for people around the world both nutritionally and culturally. In fact, the earliest archaeological example of cheese production is a ceramic cheese drain mold, found in Poland and dating from 7,500 years ago, complete with holes providing drainage for the whey, a byproduct of the cheesemaking process. When archaeologists analyzed the ceramic, they found evidence that milk fats and lipids had stuck in its pores. Traditional cultures continue to safely access raw milk; remember the Samburu in this book's introduction, who mixed fresh milk with cow's blood as a source of easily sustainable, portable, high-quality nutrition. And in Chapter 8, I'll take you to the lowlands of Kenya to see how fermented, clabbered milk and ash are used to make the yogurt called mursik.

For the most part, though, these traditional technologies and processes aren't quick. They're labor- and time-intensive. And, as we've seen with other foods that had been safely consumed for ages when processed using traditional technologies (maize, for example), much to our detriment we left these tried-and-true methods behind as population and milk demand grew. The swill dairies of the mid-1800s in the United States present one of the most egregious examples. Conceived as a way to maximize profits, these dairies were established next to distilleries so that cows could be fed the grain mash (swill) left over from alcohol production. Kept in miserable, filthy conditions and fed unnatural waste products, these cows produced bluish, foul milk that the producers doctored with everything from molasses to plaster of Paris to animal brains for a more natural appearance, creamy top, and thick consistency. Then, they marketed it as country-fresh milk, sickening and killing thousands who consumed it. The *New York Times* attributed 8,000 deaths a year—mostly children—to this milk, causing an understandable national uproar and a push toward better regulation of milk. By the 1920s, officials implemented a new technology called pasteurization, which uses heat to kill off pathogens and bacteria in milk and to increase its shelf life. This process became widespread by the 1950s, according to the Centers for Disease Control (CDC), making the mass-produced milk on our grocery store shelves uniformly safe for consumption.

Nevertheless, misconceptions about milk—whether pasteurized or raw—continue to damage our relationship with this fundamental food. From the 1970s through the '90s, governmental dietary regulations, nutritionists, and doctors cautioned against consuming whole milk, linking its high saturated fat content to obesity, heart disease, and a host of other contemporary Western ills. Their answer was to skim most of the fat off milk and then homogenize what remained, removing any need for consumers to deal with a layer of cream (fat) on the milk. Today, federal food guidelines continue to recommend low-fat or nonfat milk as part of our diet, demonizing the healthy fats that exist in whole milk and cream. Meanwhile, the CDC starkly warns against using raw milk on its website, attributing 1,909 illnesses and 144 hospitalizations to raw milk consumption between 1993 and 2012, and stating that of all the foods that can make you sick, "raw milk is one of the riskiest of all." All-out battles against unadulterated, unpasteurized raw milk continue all over the world. Perhaps nowhere is this more extreme than in the US, where armed government raids on small dairy operations have resulted in arrests, fines, and the loss of multigenerational family farms simply because the farmers offered fresh milk to their customers who wanted what they considered the healthiest food they could obtain for their families.

I am not going to argue that efforts to make milk and dairy products safer through pasteurization are somehow a bad thing. There's no question that as the dairy industry moved to mass production of milk and dairy products, the labor-intensive, time-consuming methods that traditional cultures and our ancestors used for generations to make milk and dairy products safe and nutritious couldn't be scaled to meet the demand. But we have to recognize that what we have created now is a kind of Frankenmilk. While authorities debate how significantly pasteurization destroys different constituents in milk, we can safely say that it destroys enzymes such as lactase and both pathogenic and friendly bacteria (including lactobacillus). It diminishes vitamins such as A, B_{12}, C, and D, so that the milk has to be artificially fortified with these vitamins. Finally, it denatures the proteins in raw milk to the point that it is difficult or, depending on the degree of pasteurization, impossible to make cheese. For example, casein, one of the proteins found in milk, will not separate into curds properly in ultra-pasteurized milk. Most modern fermented dairy products — such as the yogurts you buy in the grocery store touting their probiotic benefits for gut health — use this pasteurized milk. To kick off the fermentation (which occurs naturally in unpasteurized milk, still full of friendly bacteria), industrial producers add lab-created bacterial colonies to mimic the ones killed through pasteurization. The act of homogenizing milk serves no real purpose other than to prevent fat from separating and cream rising to the top, so that we don't have to make the herculean effort of shaking a carton of milk before using it.

Early on in my efforts to source raw milk when I first moved to Maryland, I was sure that this heavily agricultural region would have ample dairy farms where I could purchase the milk. I was profoundly mistaken, and in one of my interviews with a prospective farmer, he scoffed at my assumption that he drank any of the milk, in any form, that his cows produced. On the contrary, he told me that his cows' milk is shipped to a central processing facility, where it is combined with milk from many other farms. There it is stripped apart, pasteurized, homogenized, and the different components recombined to meet minimum governmental standards. Finally, depending on the desired ultimate product, it is artificially fortified with any number of additives, stabilizers, vitamins, sweeteners, and/or flavorings. The finished containers of Frankenmilk are then sold in grocery stores in Virginia. He went on to tell me that his family — despite living on one of the largest dairy farms in our region — consumes milk that comes from cows in Virginia and is purchased in Maryland grocery stores! In the end, I had to find an Amish farmer in Pennsylvania who was willing to sell me raw milk. Before we started purchasing milk from him, Christina, the kids, and I spent time at his farm, talking with him and his family and seeing firsthand how they cared for their animals and maintained safety protocols for their milk. Not only did this time and effort give me peace of mind about buying milk from this farmer, it kindled a fulfilling personal relationship and ensured that we had as direct a connection as possible to our food.

Still, I understand that for some people, raw milk is too far a stretch from their comfort zone — not to mention that where I live, at least, it's illegal. I'm not going to insist that you must consume and use only raw milk in your own diet; instead, I'll give you suggestions in the tips section for how to find and use the next best thing. But what I am unequivocally stating is that our ancestors successfully used, and traditional cultures continue to use, natural fermentation technologies to turn raw, unprocessed milk into a wide array of nourishing, safe, sustainable foods, and it's entirely within your grasp to do the same in your own kitchen.

For me, this takes its finest form in cheese, deeply embedded in the Italian side of my family. My father could never resist his provolone, a trait that he has passed on to me. I can still remember the cheese platters central to family functions and my father calling out, "Provolone, sleep alone!" as he and I downed cube after cube. Some of my fondest childhood memories are of preparing eggplant parmesan with my Italian grandmother, Teresa, and the gorgeous, flavorful grilled cheese sandwiches my maternal grandmother, Granny, would make us. These were thick slices of hearty bread slathered with rich butter on the outside, and mayonnaise with a bit of curry powder and plenty of aged cheddar cheese on the inside. They bore no resemblance to the sandwiches my friends' parents made of Wonder Bread, margarine, and sliced American "cheese." Granny's sandwich had character.

In short, I love cheese, but when I started to explore how best to make it, I ran into a brick wall. While wild fermentations, using only naturally occurring yeasts and bacteria in our environments, seemed to work with everything else I was making — from sourdough to alcohol — I could find no information about using them to make cheese. It was baffling. Every recipe required me to purchase freeze-dried cultures, dozens of them specific to different types of cheeses and available from only a handful of cheesemaking equipment suppliers. I also had to buy rennet, the key ingredient for cheesemaking, and this supply chain perplexed me, too. Rennet, also known as the enzyme chymosin, is produced naturally in calves' stomachs, so you would think that there would be plenty of rennet available in this dairy system. But the reality is that when male calves are slaughtered for veal, their stomachs are tossed away as unusable, like so many of the nutrient-dense parts of animals processed in our modern system. The only option for most cheesemakers is to purchase rennet. The vast majority of this rennet is made from veal calves that are slaughtered in New Zealand. Their stomachs are shipped to Austria for processing, then the rennet is sold around the world in powder, liquid, and paste forms. Nothing in this system made sense to me. Where did the cheesemakers of our past, without access to commercially available freeze-dried cultures, obtain the bacteria with which to make their cheese? Where was the wild fermentation for dairy?

I found the answer in the oddest of places: standing in a potato storage room next to a coffee shop/pottery studio, about a two-hour drive from Reykjavík, Iceland. I'd come here to take a five-day traditional cheesemaking course with "guerrilla cheesemaker" David Asher, author of *The Art of Natural Cheesemaking: Using Traditional, Non-Industrial Methods and Raw Ingredients to Make the World's Best Cheeses*. The course drew participants from all over the world, including the United States, Canada, Iceland, Ireland, and Kenya. After days of study, we had taken the step of seeking cheese at its original source, inside the fourth stomach chamber — the abomasum — of a freshly killed veal calf. As with human babies, when a calf feeds from its mother, the milk coming from her is full of beneficial bacteria and already in the process of fermenting. In the act of stretching its neck, the calf positions its digestive tract so that the milk flows directly to this fourth stomach, bypassing the others, which are still developing at this stage. When the milk reaches the fourth stomach, it comes in contact with chymosin, the enzyme that coagulates, or curdles, the milk and helps it stay in the calf's digestive tract longer, where it continues to ferment and chemically and physically break down, enabling the young animal to access all of its nutrients. Once we removed the abomasum, we realized that it was full, and most of the contents were semi-solid; this was, essentially, the most original form of cheese. After straining the contents (and taking a small sample to taste), we washed out the stomach and covered it in salt to begin the curing process. What remained in the strainer was the cheese the calf's stomach had produced naturally.

At that moment, I felt a profound connection to the past. It was easy to see how one of our ancestors could have put two and two together when they witnessed this phenomenon after butchering a young animal and seeing the contents of its stomach. They would have realized that there was something special about that stomach, and perhaps all they needed to do was place a piece of it or some of its contents in fresh milk and replicate the process outside the animal's body. Raw milk's natural microorganisms would spur the fermentation, and they could separate the curds and whey using the rennet from the animal's stomach, and control variables during the fermentation and aging stages to produce different results. The specific ways in which various cultures over time accomplished this produced the wide variety of cheeses around the world. As just one example, Italy has more than 350 different types of cheeses subdivided into about 1,000 varieties.

The same is true for our process today. To replicate what happens naturally in a calf's stomach, all you need is rennet, milk, salt, and a cheese-making vessel — a pot or bowl — that essentially substitutes for the calf's stomach. The first step is to heat milk — ideally raw milk — in a pot on the stove and maintain a temperature of approximately 100°F (close to a calf's body temperature). If you don't have access to raw milk, you'll need to add a colony of live, beneficial bacteria cultures to your pasteurized milk to kick-start its fermentation. You can do this by adding kefir (at a ratio of approximately 2 percent kefir to 100 percent milk) or freeze-dried cheesemaking cultures made especially for this purpose, found online at cheesemaking supply shops. To the fermenting milk you simply add rennet, which in turn coagulates the milk, similar to what happens in a calf's stomach, forming what is called a curd. Once the curd takes on the consistency of Jell-O, it is set, and with this you have the most basic form of cheese. Serious cheesemakers will then cut this curd with a knife to separate the curds from the whey and control for nuances such as time, temperature, humidity, curd size, and pressure to produce everything from soft, milky chèvre to hard, tangy Parmesan.

As is typical of the modern food system, of course, some cheesemakers have found shortcuts that bypass the traditional process. Perhaps the worst shortcut happens with mozzarella. Do you know someone who is lactose intolerant but can eat a high-quality mozzarella without any issues? This is because traditional mozzarella requires about eight hours to reach the necessary pH (5.2) to stretch it. To cut this process short, some cheesemakers use vinegar or lactic acid to alter the pH, speeding up the process by bypassing the time needed for fermentation. But in bypassing fermentation, they are leaving the lactose intact. The final product may look and taste the same, but if you're lactose intolerant, you'll immediately know the difference. Here's the easy way to spot "fake" mozzarella: Read the ingredients. All that real mozzarella should contain is milk, rennet, and salt. It will also contain live active cultures or bacteria, unless it is made from raw milk, with nothing acidic added. "Fake" mozzarella will contain vinegar, lactic acid, or citric acid. If you find these on the label, it is not real cheese.

Additionally, many products on our grocery store shelves contain the word *cheese* on their labels but are nothing like traditional cheese made from high-quality, fermented milk. The FDA-defined categories of processed cheese, processed cheese food, processed cheese spread, processed cheese products, and imitation cheese are all made with additives, emulsifiers, chemicals, and industrial processes. You should avoid them since they have not gone through the fermentation process to render the product safe for those with lactose intolerance, nor do they deliver the same nutrition as traditionally produced cheese.

Some people will continue to argue that as our bodies naturally outgrow the need for — and even tolerance of — the milk that sustained us as infants, we should eliminate it from our diets. I would argue that we should instead rethink and refine our relationship with this most fundamental of foods. Wild fermentation of dairy increases its shelf life, taste, texture, and smell; we love the creaminess of butter, the sharpness of cheese, and the sourness of yogurt. More importantly, it supercharges milk's health benefits, boosting its nutrient density and the strength and quantity of beneficial bacteria and probiotics, while decreasing the sugar lactose. In fact, when fermented long enough, lactose nearly disappears; that's why someone who's lactose intolerant can eat aged cheeses but can't safely drink a glass of pasteurized milk. And you don't need a three-year-old cheddar to do this. Even yogurt that has been cultured for 24 hours has consumed all of its lactose.

There is no reason you cannot accomplish these fermentations in your own kitchen to produce delicious, healthful butters, cheeses, and yogurts. The single most important thing to remember is to start with the cleanest and freshest source of milk possible. Ideally, this is raw milk, but if you have access only to pasteurized milk, don't worry; you can still use the techniques in this book to restore it to something alive, nutrient-dense, and full of most of the same health benefits as a fermented raw milk product — what cheese expert David Asher calls "un-pasteurizing." Ideally, if you have access to fresh raw milk, you will create a clabber culture, which is simply raw milk left to ferment at room temperature. You can then keep this going as the source of bacteria not just to inoculate milk to make a number of different cheeses but also to inoculate cream to make crème fraîche and butter. I keep three dairy cultures going at the same time — a clabber culture, a kefir culture, and an heirloom yogurt culture. This may be a little extreme, but the reality is it takes only a few minutes once or twice a week to tend to these cultures, and the variety they provide is truly limitless. When I refresh them, I throw the leftovers into a blender with fresh fruit and sometimes a little honey to produce a shake for the kids' breakfast that they look forward to every week. I would suggest that you always make your own yogurt, kefir, and butter; you simply cannot purchase anything at the market that is as good as what you can produce at home. And while cheese is my passion, I understand that you may not have the time or inclination to produce all the cheese that your family might consume, especially with an increasing diversity of excellent local cheese producers. That said, making cheese even once and understanding the process can help you make better choices at the supermarket and support those cheese producers who are doing it right.

TIPS AND RECIPES

HOW TO BUY MILK

The dairy aisles in our grocery stores today contain hundreds of different products — everything, it seems, except the milk our ancestors consumed. Following is my guide for making the healthiest choices, with healthiest on top. Milk labeled A2, which you can find at most health food stores as well as larger supermarkets, is a good option. The A2 protein makes the milk more digestible for humans. Try not to drink any milk that is ultra-pasteurized.

1. If it's legal in your state, high-quality, raw, unpasteurized whole milk from a small, grass-fed dairy where you know the farmer and the farmer knows you. *If you don't know anything about the source, do not buy raw milk.* Here's a great source to find raw milk: realmilk.com/real-milk-finder.
2. Low-temperature pasteurized, non-homogenized, organic whole milk from a small dairy.
3. Pasteurized, non-homogenized, organic whole milk.
4. Pasteurized, homogenized, organic whole milk.

Recommended Equipment for Fermenting Dairy

Stainless steel, glass, or plastic bowls of various sizes (do not use aluminum as it will react negatively with the low pH of the fermenting dairy)

Quart-size mason jars

Cheesecloth or butter muslin (cheesecloth is meant for single use, while butter muslin can be reused)

Stainless steel or plastic colanders and sieves of various sizes

Instant-read digital thermometer, preferably waterproof

Optional Equipment for Fermenting Dairy

Ricotta drain mold (available from cheesemaking supply companies online)

Kitchen scale

Yogurt maker, dehydrator, sous vide immersion circulator, or small cooler

A Note About Rennet

Many of the recipes in this chapter require rennet. You can choose to use animal, vegetable, or microbial rennet to make your cheese. I use animal rennet in all of my cheesemaking. This is a conscious decision because it is traditional and provides the best results, and from a philosophical perspective, it makes me feel I am a step closer to a process that our ancestors have used for generations. Rennet can be found at online cheesemaking supply sources such as thecheesemaker.com.

KEFIR

Kefir is the easiest dairy fermentation to do without any special equipment and with milk you can buy off the grocery store shelf. Get the freshest, highest-quality organic milk available; raw is best, but pasteurized is okay (ultra-pasteurized will not work). Kefir grains, added to milk, introduce the beneficial bacteria needed for fermentation. It is best to use utensils made of plastic or stainless steel because other metals will react negatively with the kefir grains. If you don't know anyone making kefir who can share starter grains, you can purchase kefir grains online at sources such as culturesforhealth.com.

2 tablespoons kefir grains
3½ cups milk

Combine the kefir grains and milk in a quart-size mason jar. Cover with a lid and leave in a warm place in your kitchen for 24 hours. Open the jar to examine the contents. The kefir should be thickened and have a pleasant, slightly yeasty and yogurty aroma. Look through the side of the jar. There should be no bubbles and no separation of whey. Now taste a small amount. It should have a very pleasant sour flavor.

Set a plastic or stainless steel strainer with large-size mesh (up to about ⅛ inch) over a bowl and pour the contents of the jar through the strainer. Use a silicone spatula to very gently coax the kefir through the strainer, making sure not to bruise or injure the kefir grains that remain behind in the strainer.

Strained kefir can be consumed right away, used as an ingredient in a variety of recipes (including as a base for the Clay Smoothie on page 239), or stored in the refrigerator for up to 2 weeks.

Note:

To make a second batch, wash the jar (this is an optional step, as many people continuously reuse the jar without washing). Put the grains back in the jar and add 3½ more cups of milk. Return to a warm location and ferment for 24 hours. Repeat daily as desired or, if you have enough kefir and want to put the process on pause, place the jar containing the kefir and grains at the end of a 24-hour fermentation session (that is, before straining) in the fridge for up to 1 week. When you are ready to begin fermenting again, remove it from the fridge, strain, refresh, and ferment as above.

MESOPHILIC YOGURT

In the 1970s, Dannon launched a massive advertising campaign to persuade Americans to start eating a strange, sour, fermented milk–based product called yogurt. This extremely successful campaign focused on the Caucasus region of what was then Soviet Georgia, which supported a markedly high number of centenarians. It suggested that their longevity was due to the prevalence of yogurt in their diet.

The yogurt of that region, matsoni, is a type of mesophilic yogurt, which means it cultures at room temperature. Since it does not need to be kept at 110°F like most other yogurts, it doesn't require any special equipment or attention to make. It is an excellent yogurt to begin with if you are just starting out.

This recipe requires an heirloom mesophilic yogurt (like matsoni) to provide the proper bacteria to activate the fermentation. If you don't already have one left over from a previous batch, you can purchase one from a reputable source such as culturesforhealth.com. You can use milk from the grocery store; get the freshest, highest-quality organic milk available. Raw is best, but pasteurized is okay (ultra-pasteurized will not work).

> 7⅔ cups milk
> ⅓ cup mesophilic yogurt

Pour the milk into a saucepan and slowly warm over low heat, making sure to stir occasionally to avoid burning the bottom or forming a skin on the top. When it reaches approximately 75°F, it is ready.

Put the yogurt in a 2-quart mason jar (or divide evenly between two 1-quart mason jars). Pour about ½ cup of the warm milk into the jar. Whisk the culture and milk together until smooth. This helps make sure the yogurt culture is evenly distributed and not chunky.

Pour the rest of the milk into the jar, stir to distribute evenly, cover, and leave in a warm place in your kitchen where it will not be disturbed. It is very important not to move the jar while the yogurt cultures. The curd is very soft as it develops, and moving it will break up the curd, releasing whey and resulting in a yogurt that is not thickened properly.

After 8 to 12 hours, check your yogurt by removing the lid and tilting the jar gently to one side. If it pulls away from the side slightly and seems thickened, it is finished. Put the lid back on and put the jar in the refrigerator. If it is not ready, continue to ferment until it is thickened. Once thickened, it is ready to eat or can be stored in the fridge for up to 2 weeks.

But remember, don't eat it all! You need to save some to make the next batch. In fact, now is a great time to reserve fresh yogurt in a separate half-pint mason jar. Keep it in the fridge clearly labeled so no one eats it and it is ready for the next time you want to make yogurt.

THERMOPHILIC YOGURT

MAKES 2 QUARTS

If you use yogurt from the grocery store to culture milk and make yogurt, you need to find a way to maintain approximately 110°F throughout the fermentation phase. Most commercially available yogurt is thermophilic, which means it ferments at a higher temperature than mesophilic. However, the bacteria in many commercial yogurts consist of lab-created colonies that cannot be sustained long-term at home.

Traditional heirloom cultures are made of natural bacterial colonies that live together harmoniously and can make yogurt over and over again indefinitely. This recipe requires an heirloom thermophilic yogurt culture to provide the proper bacteria to activate the fermentation. If you don't already have one left over from a previous batch, you can purchase one from a reputable source like culturesforhealth.com. You can use milk from the grocery store; get the freshest, highest-quality organic milk available. Raw is best, but pasteurized is okay (ultra-pasteurized will not work).

7⅔ cups milk
⅓ cup thermophilic yogurt

Pour the milk into a saucepan and slowly warm over low heat. If you are using raw milk and want to keep it raw, only heat it until it reaches 110°F. Otherwise, continue to heat the milk until it reaches 180°F, stirring constantly to avoid burning the bottom or forming a skin on the top. While the milk is heating, prepare an ice-water bath in your sink or in a bowl large enough to accommodate the cooking vessel. Once the milk has reached 180°F, place the pot in the ice bath and continue to stir until the temperature drops to 110°F.

Put the yogurt in a 2-quart mason jar (or divide evenly between two 1-quart mason jars). Pour about ½ cup of the warm milk into the jar.

Whisk the culture and milk together until smooth. This helps make sure the yogurt culture is evenly distributed and not chunky.

Pour the rest of the milk into the jar, stir to distribute evenly, cover, and maintain at 110°F in a location where it will not be disturbed. There are several ways to maintain the necessary temperature. Common methods include using a commercial yogurt maker or placing it in a large food dehydrator (such as an Excalibur with the shelves removed), in a water bath with a sous vide immersion circulator, or in a cooler filled with 110°F water to just below the rim of the jar. It is very important not to move the jar while it cultures. The curd is very soft as it develops, and moving it will break up the curd, releasing whey and resulting in a yogurt that is not thickened properly.

After 8 to 12 hours, check your yogurt by removing the lid and tilting the jar gently to one side. If it pulls away from the side slightly and seems thickened, it is finished. Put the lid back on and put the jar in the refrigerator. If it is not ready, continue to ferment for several more hours at 110°F until it's thickened. Once thickened, it is ready to eat or can be stored in the fridge for up to 2 weeks.

But remember, don't eat it all! You need to save some to make the next batch. In fact, now is a great time to reserve fresh yogurt in a separate half-pint mason jar. Keep it in the fridge clearly labeled so no one eats it and it is ready for the next time you want to make yogurt.

FERMENTED CREAM (CRÈME FRAÎCHE, CREMA)

When made traditionally, fermented cream is a delicious, nourishing, alive, probiotic food. It is easy to make and versatile in the kitchen, lending flavor, aroma, and nutrition to savory and sweet dishes. Use it on top of tacos, as an ingredient in blue cheese dressing, or even served with fruit. Making fermented cream is also the first step in making Fermented Butter (page 189). I typically double this recipe and churn half for butter and keep the other half in a mason jar in the fridge.

You can use cream from the grocery store; get the freshest, highest-quality organic cream available. Raw is best, but pasteurized is okay (ultra-pasteurized will not work). If you don't have leftover kefir or mesophilic yogurt to use as your starter, you can purchase some from a reputable source such as culturesforhealth.com.

1 quart heavy cream
2 tablespoons Kefir (page 181), Mesophilic Yogurt (page 183), or
  thermophilic yogurt in a pinch

Pour the cream into a saucepan and slowly warm over low heat, making sure to stir occasionally to avoid burning on the bottom or forming a skin on the top. When it reaches approximately 75°F, it is ready.

Put the kefir or yogurt in a quart-size mason jar. Pour about ½ cup of the warm cream into the jar. Whisk the culture and cream together until smooth. This helps make sure the culture is evenly distributed. Pour the rest of the cream into the jar, stir to distribute, cover, and leave in a warm place in your kitchen where it will not be disturbed for 12 to 24 hours. It is very important not to move the jar while the cream cultures.

After 12 hours, use a small spoon to scoop a little out of the jar. It should have thickened to the point where the impression made by the spoon remains. Now taste it. It should have a wonderful, slightly sour taste and a complex aroma. If you are happy with its consistency and taste, cover and transfer to the refrigerator, or use it to make Fermented Butter (page 189). If you would like the cream thicker or want it to develop more flavor, cover and set in a warm place to continue to ferment for up to another 12 hours. Store covered in the refrigerator for up to 2 weeks.

FERMENTED BUTTER

Before refrigeration, butter was naturally a fermented food. Farmers would milk their cows, collect the milk, and let it sit until the fat separated and floated to the top. This cream was collected and set aside, because butter-making by hand is laborious, and it didn't make sense to churn butter with only a little cream. Each day more cream would be skimmed and added. Eventually, days later, the farmer had collected enough cream to make butter. Because the milk and cream were raw and there was no refrigeration, the cream was fermenting the entire time.

Fermenting cream before it is made into butter offers several advantages. First, the act of churning the butter physically breaks down the membrane on the outside of the fat globules so that they come together to form the mass of butter. Fermenting helps to chemically break down the membrane so that it's easier and quicker to churn. Fermenting also improves the flavor, lowers the pH to create a safer environment, and increases the probiotic content of the butter.

If you're not using a stand mixer, see the note below for instructions on how to mix by hand.

1 quart Fermented Cream (page 187)
½ teaspoon sea salt (optional)

Pour the cultured cream into the bowl of a stand mixer fitted with the whisk attachment, making sure to fill it no more than halfway. The cream will expand as it fills with air, and you need to leave room for the expansion. If your mixer has a splash guard, by all means use it. When the buttermilk first separates from the butterfat, the mixture becomes unbalanced and splashes everywhere. Some people even wrap their entire machine with a towel to avoid the mess, and I don't blame them.

Turn on your mixer at the lowest speed. Slowly increase the speed until you are whisking at one of the highest speeds. Find the happy medium that allows you to whisk at a high speed without spraying fermented cream all over the kitchen. Watch it closely. After a few minutes, the cream will go through different stages, from cream to whipped cream to separating into butter and buttermilk. You can tell it is about to separate when you see the small pearls of butter emerging. As soon as they are visible, immediately reduce the speed to its lowest setting; otherwise you'll be cleaning up the mess for hours. Continue to whisk at a low speed for an additional 30 seconds or so. This helps expel a little more of the buttermilk and makes the rest of the process easier.

Remove the whisk and use a silicone spatula to scrape off as much butter clinging to it as possible. Place a large bowl in the sink and set a large sieve or colander lined with cheesecloth or butter muslin in it. Using the spatula, scrape the contents of the mixing bowl into the colander, allowing the buttermilk to drain into the bowl. Pour the collected buttermilk into a jar, cover, and refrigerate. This can be used immediately or refrigerated for up to 1 week.

All of the remaining buttermilk must be removed to prolong the butter's shelf life. Hold the sieve containing the butterfat and residual buttermilk under the faucet and let cold water pass through. This washes away much of the residual buttermilk and chills the butterfat, making it firmer and easier to handle. Once you have sufficiently rinsed the butter, transfer it to a large bowl. Fill the bowl with fresh cold water. Using the spatula or your hands, repeatedly fold the butter onto itself, squeezing out any remaining buttermilk. As the buttermilk is released, it will cloud the water. When that happens, pour out the water, add fresh, and repeat until the water stays clear.

If desired, sprinkle the salt on the butter, fold to combine, taste, and adjust if necessary. Salting increases the shelf life by drawing out moisture. Let the salted butter sit in the bowl for about 15 minutes. Pour off any liquid that has accumulated at the bottom of the bowl and pat the butter dry. Transfer the butter to a covered container and store at room temperature for several days, or to a butter bell for a couple of weeks. Or, wrap it in wax paper, parchment, or an airtight container to refrigerate for several weeks or freeze for several months.

Note:

If you do not have a stand mixer, a hand mixer or food processor will work fine. If you are looking for a workout, you can even make butter by shaking in a jar! To do this, you'll need a jar that is large enough so it's only two-thirds full of fermented cream, to allow space for the contents to slam against the top and bottom of the jar when it is shaken. You might need to use less cream if you don't have a large enough jar. Make sure the lid is on tightly, and shake the jar up and down until the butterfat separates from the buttermilk. Depending on the quantity of cream, degree of fermentation, and vigorousness of shaking, this may take as long as 30 minutes.

MOZZARELLA

You can easily make high-quality cheese in your own home kitchen. If you think it is out of your reach, just remember that our ancestors made cheese for thousands of years using nothing but clay pots, an open fire, and drain molds woven out of reeds.

This recipe is for mozzarella or, more accurately, fior di latte, "flower of milk." Mozzarella is technically made from buffalo milk, while fior di latte is made from cow's milk. Both are members of a very interesting family of cheeses called pasta filata. This stretched-curd cheese begins as almost any real cheese does: with fermentation. The milk begins to ferment because either it is raw or it is inoculated with an outside source of bacteria. Inoculation methods include exposure to cheesemaking equipment with the previous batch's remnants still adhering to the surface or trapped within its pores; intentional introduction of bacteria from whey left over from the cheesemaking process; or use of kefir, yogurt, clabber, or a freeze-dried culture containing an isolated strain of bacteria designed for the specific cheese desired.

The way we cut and heat the curds in this recipe results in a low-moisture, firmer cheese than you would expect from a ball of fresh mozzarella. This is intentional. Other than simply slicing and eating with tomatoes and basil, fresh mozzarella is not very practical, nor does it store well. This version, on the other hand, is more versatile. It can be eaten fresh, melted, and even frozen for long-term storage. Once you have created the curd and taken it through the fermentation process, you can use different techniques to stretch it into a variety of fun and delicious cheeses, such as Quesillo (page 201) and String Cheese (page 200).

You can use milk from the grocery store for this recipe; get the freshest, highest-quality organic milk available. Raw is best, but pasteurized is okay (ultra-pasteurized will not work). This recipe assumes you are using pasteurized milk and thus will require the addition of kefir or another culture to introduce the live bacteria needed to kick-start the fermentation. You could also use live whey or, even better, clabber if you have access to it. Use freeze-dried cultures as a last resort. They are expensive and unnecessary, and have little place in a kitchen where reconnecting with our food and dietary past is a priority.

One final word before we get started: There is a 30-minute mozzarella recipe that can be found all over the internet. It relies on vinegar, lemon juice, or citric acid to drop the pH and arrive at the required 5.2 to stretch. Avoid it. It is akin to making a yeasted bread instead of sourdough or vinegar pickles instead of lacto-fermented ones. The final product may superficially resemble the authentic version, but it pales in comparison in terms of flavor and nutritional value. Plus, for those who suffer from lactose intolerance, this shortcut version is the same as drinking a glass of milk since all of the lactose remains in the final product.

> 1 gallon milk
> ⅓ cup Kefir (page 181), Thermophilic Yogurt (page 185), or a freeze-dried thermophilic culture (follow the manufacturer's instructions for quantity)
> ¼ cup cold water
> Rennet (liquid, powder, or tablet form — follow the manufacturer's instructions for quantity)
> Sea salt

Step 1: Fermenting the Milk and Creating the Curd

Pour the milk into a heavy-bottomed pot and warm over very low heat to slowly bring the milk to approximately 100°F, stirring occasionally to ensure the bottom does not burn and a skin does not form on the top. Turn off the heat.

If using kefir or yogurt, pour it into a medium bowl. Transfer about 1 cup of the warm milk to the bowl and whisk until smooth. Return the mixture to the pot of milk and stir to combine.

If using a freeze-dried culture, refer to the package to determine how much is needed. Sprinkle the measured amount evenly across the top of the milk in the pot, allow it to hydrate undisturbed for 5 minutes, then stir to distribute evenly throughout the milk.

Allow the milk to sit in the pot, covered, for approximately 1 hour to begin fermenting.

After the hour has passed, pour the cold water into a small bowl. Add the required amount of rennet for 1 gallon of milk (follow the manufacturer's instructions, as doses vary by type and strength of the rennet). If the rennet is in powder or tablet form, allow it to fully dissolve in the water, then stir. Using a spoon, begin to stir the warmed milk to get it moving in a whirlpool-like motion. Add the rennet mixture as you continue to stir. Rennet is powerful and must be evenly distributed as quickly as possible before it begins to set the curd. Cover the pot and let it sit, undisturbed, for 30 to 60 minutes.

Step 2: Cutting the Curd

After 30 minutes, use the tip of a sharp knife to cut a small piece of curd out of the thickened mass, leaving a small divot behind. Take note of the edges of the divot. If the edges of the cut section remain fairly sharp, then you are ready to cut the curd. If they become round quickly and/or the divot you created disappears, it needs more time. Check it every 15 minutes until it is ready.

Cut the curds aggressively with a whisk until they are the size of rice grains. Turn the heat to medium-low and stir continuously with a spoon, making sure that the curds do not stick to the bottom of the pot or clump together, until the liquid (whey) reaches a temperature of approximately 120°F. Turn off the heat and let the curds settle to the bottom of the pot, undisturbed, for 15 minutes.

Step 3: Separating the Curds and Whey

Use a small bowl or ladle to remove as much whey as possible and transfer it to another container. It is important to keep from disturbing the bed of cheese curds at the bottom of the pot. It helps to use the back side of a sieve, colander, or cheese drain mold to hold the curds in place while you ladle out the whey — or "whey off," as it is referred to in the cheese-making world.

Line a colander with cheesecloth and set it in a large bowl. Use a cheese drain mold, sieve, small colander, or slotted spoon to transfer the curds to the colander. Fold the ends of the cheesecloth over the top and place the cheesecloth and curds back in the pot. Gently pour some of the whey back into the pot, ensuring that the curds are completely submerged. The whey at this point is considered "sweet whey" since it has not fermented for too long. You only need enough whey to just cover the curds, so use any remaining whey to make your saturated brine (see below) or Ricotta (page 203). (Unless you are making a huge quantity of cheese, you will not have enough whey left over to make both the brine and the ricotta. Once you have made the brine, it can be stored in the fridge for several weeks and reused. After that you can use the whey the next time you make ricotta.)

The curds will take between 4 and 8 hours to ferment to the point that they are ready to stretch. During this time, the curds and whey need to remain at body temperature, about 100°F. Check them periodically and add a few cups of warm water to the whey as needed to maintain temperature.

Step 4: Making the Saturated Brine

Once you stretch and shape your mozzarella, you will immediately place the warm cheese into a brine to cool, firm up, and absorb salt. The best brine for this cheese is a saturated brine, which simply means it is holding the maximum amount of salt in solution as possible (26 percent). The amount of salt required can be calculated by multiplying the weight of the whey by 0.26. If you do not have a scale, add ¼ cup salt to room-temperature whey and stir. Continue adding ¼ cup salt at a time, stirring between additions, until salt accumulates at the bottom of the container, indicating the solution is "saturated." If you do not have enough whey to make a brine in which you can fully submerge four fist-size balls of cheese, you can make a suitable brine using a combination of water and whey or just water. Once made, the brine can be stored in the fridge, covered, for several weeks.

Step 5: Testing the Curds

Once the curds have been fermenting for 4 hours, heat water to 180°F. Slice off a piece of curd about 1 inch square and ⅛ inch thick. Put it in a medium bowl and add enough of the hot water to cover the curd. Let the curd warm for a minute or two, then use a spoon to pull it out of the water. If it is ready, you should be able to see it stretch. Grab one end of the warmed curd and lift it off the spoon. If it stretches easily into long threads without breaking, it is ready for the next step (see Figure 1). If it breaks easily, it needs more time to ferment. Continue checking every 30 minutes until it passes the test.

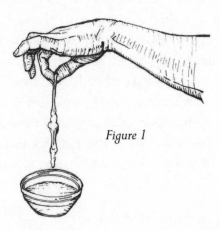

Figure 1

Step 6: Stretching the Curds

Heat water to 180°F. Cut the curd into quarters with a knife. Slice one portion into ¼-inch-thick slices and put them in a medium bowl. Pour some of the hot water down along the side of the bowl (not directly on the curds) until the curds are submerged. Wait a few minutes for the curds to begin to warm.

Using a spoon, gently move the curd slices around until they begin to come together as one solid mass (see Figure 2). Pull the mass out of the water, stretch it slightly, fold it over itself, and return it to the water. Once it's warmed again, pull it out of the water again, stretch, fold, and return to the hot water. Repeat this several times to ensure that the chunks of curd become incorporated into the solid, silky, shiny mass. Be careful not to overwork the cheese; this will toughen it and dry it out. If at any time during this process the water immersing the curds has cooled, gently tilt the bowl to pour off the water, carefully leaving the curds undisturbed, and add more hot water.

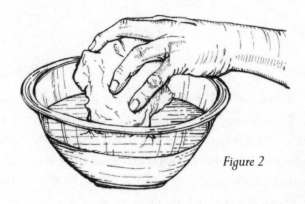

Figure 2

Once you are confident the mass is uniformly smooth, pull it out of the water, stretch, and fold it over itself into thirds (see Figure 3). Starting at the top of the curd mass, with your thumb and forefinger together, bring your hand down around the ball, separating your thumb and forefinger as you descend and stretching the cheese to form a skin around the ball. When you reach the bottom of the ball, curl your forefinger into a tight circle, bringing your thumb tightly around your forefinger as if you are making an overly tight "OK" sign (see Figure 4). Pinch the cheese closed with your fingers; the pressure and residual heat should weld the ends together.

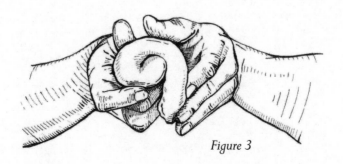

Figure 3

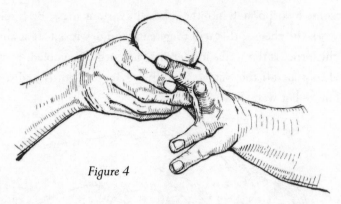

Figure 4

Finally, release the ball of cheese from the little bit of cheese remaining in your clenched fingers by tearing it. *Mozzarella* comes from the Italian word *mozzare,* which means to "cut off," and it refers to this action. Place the ball of cheese in the saturated whey brine and allow it to cool and brine for 2 hours. Repeat the stretching process to form balls from the remaining three portions of curd, and add them to the brine.

Once it is brined, the mozzarella can be eaten fresh or stored, wrapped tightly or in an airtight container, in the refrigerator for up to 1 week or in the freezer for several months.

STRACCIATELLA

This cheese is easy to make and a delicious way to use leftover mozzarella. It makes a great addition to a cheese board, can be paired with fresh tomatoes and sourdough bread, or can even be served as a side dish for dinner. *Stracciare* means "to tear" in Italian, and you make this cheese by pulling or tearing cheese (just as you would string cheese) and adding cream. This recipe uses fermented cream to boost nutrition and flavor.

   1 fist-size ball Mozzarella (page 192)
   1 cup Fermented Cream (page 187)

Pull the mozzarella into fine threads and put them in a bowl. Add the fermented cream and stir to combine. Serve immediately or store in an airtight container in the refrigerator for up to 1 week. Make sure to bring the stracciatella to room temperature before serving.

STRING CHEESE

Makes about 12 sticks

These are an excellent addition to your kid's lunch box or as a go-to snack. Since you are making them from scratch, you control the quality of the milk that goes into them, and you're using a traditional cheesemaking process to transform that milk into the most nourishing and delicious cheese sticks possible.

> 8 ounces mozzarella cheese curd ready to be stretched
> Saturated brine

Follow the directions in the recipe for mozzarella through Step 5 (page 196). Slice and heat the cheese curd with hot (180°F) water as in the mozzarella recipe. But instead of stretching the curd into the shape of a ball, stretch it into a long rope approximately ¾ inch in diameter. Cut the rope into pieces 4 or 5 inches long and let sit in the saturated brine for 10 to 15 minutes to cool and absorb the salt. Remove from the brine, pat dry, and store in the fridge in an airtight container for up to 1 week.

QUESILLO (OAXACAN STRING CHEESE)

Contrary to popular belief, cheddar cheese has no business inside of a taco or quesadilla. Traditionally, a Mexican version of pasta filata cheese, quesillo (aka Oaxacan string cheese), is used. This cheese is typically made in a long, thin ribbon, salted, and then wound like yarn into a beautiful ball. These impressive balls of coiled cheese are common throughout the markets in Oaxaca, where you can buy the cheese by the ball or by length. To use, uncoil a strip of cheese, tear it off, then shred it into finer threads (as you would with Stracciatella—see page 199). This step is necessary because the texture of the cheese is a crucial part of the overall eating experience. These threads can be eaten as is or used in quesadillas or on top of tacos.

1 cup kosher salt
1 pound mozzarella cheese curd ready to be stretched

Pour the salt into a rimmed baking sheet next to the bowl where you will be working the curd.

Follow the directions in the recipe for mozzarella through Step 5 (page 196). Divide the cheese curd into four equal portions. Working with one at a time, slice and heat the cheese curd with hot (180°F) water according to Step 6 in the mozzarella recipe (page 196). Stretch, fold, and work to ensure the chunks of curd are incorporated into a solid, silky, shiny mass. Once you are confident the mass is uniformly smooth, stretch it into one long ribbon approximately 1 inch wide. Add the ribbon to the baking sheet with the salt and, using your hands, coat the ribbon evenly. Whatever sticks to it is the ideal amount.

Starting at one end, begin to wrap the ribbon around itself as if you were winding a ball of yarn. When you reach the end, tuck it inside a coil to secure. Place the ball in a bowl to finish cooling so that it retains its shape. Repeat the stretching process to form balls from the remaining three portions of curd, and add them to the bowl. Use immediately or wrap tightly and store in the fridge for up to 1 week.

RICOTTA

The two primary proteins in milk are casein and whey protein. The casein is removed from the whey during the cheesemaking process to form the curd. However, the whey protein still remains in the whey, and this is what ricotta cheese in Italy—and its counterpart in Mexico, requeson—are made from. *Ricotta* literally means "to recook" in Italian, and *requeson* means "to remake the cheese" in Spanish.

These cheeses were traditionally made by allowing the whey left over from making pasta filata cheese to ferment a little longer to achieve a pH of about 5.9, then heating it to almost boiling to release the whey curds. These are skimmed off and drained in special drain molds or cheesecloth. Ricotta cheese is versatile and can be eaten fresh, baked to make ricotta al forno, or even dried and salted to make ricotta salata.

> 2 quarts fresh whey left over from making Mozzarella
> (see Step 4 on page 195)
> 1 cup milk
> 1 cup water
> 1 tablespoon sea salt

Combine all the ingredients in a large pot and mix well. Slowly heat to approximately 200°F without stirring unless absolutely necessary to prevent burning. The ricotta curds are fragile, and disturbing them can affect the final product. When the curds—which will look like soft, fluffy cottage cheese—accumulate at the top, turn off the heat and allow to sit for 15 minutes before skimming and placing the curds in ricotta drain molds or a colander lined with cheesecloth. If you reach 200°F and the curds have not accumulated at the top, the pH may not be low enough. In that case add 1 tablespoon apple cider vinegar or lemon juice and stir gently. If curds still do not appear, repeat until they do, then drain as directed above.

The ricotta can be used immediately or refrigerated in a covered container for up to 1 week.

Chapter 7

BUGS

PROTEIN, NOT PESTS

I did my best to smile as I watched my 10-year-old daughter, Alyssa, dive into the trio of rainbow-colored waffles on her plate. Accompanying the waffles were slices of bananas and strawberries, marshmallows, whipped cream, and three equally colorful scoops of ice cream, which were topped with cones, pointy end up. It was a spectacular, if overwrought, presentation, but I couldn't deny that the upside-down ice-cream cones did indeed look like unicorn horns.

And unicorns were what it was all about at the Unicorn Cafe in Bangkok, Thailand.

I've eaten all kinds of weird foods in wild places but never experienced anything like that. Unicorns exploded across the restaurant's artwork, tables, and food—all in glittery pastel shades of pink, blue, lavender, and peach. Unicorn galaxy paintings and rainbow-colored paper adorned the walls, while an eclectic array of pink, blue, and gold plush furniture, studded with fake gems, was scattered about. Stuffed unicorns hanging from the ceiling galloped over our heads, and as we waited for our food to arrive, we could snuggle with more stuffed unicorns and even don a unicorn onesie as our dining attire (adult or child size). I had told Alyssa I'd do this with her—yes, wear a unicorn onesie—but she was too embarrassed to wear one and definitely too embarrassed to have her father wear one.

No matter, a deal's a deal, and as a parent I'm not above bribery. In this case, I had agreed a few weeks earlier that when we went to Thailand to explore insects as food, *if* Alyssa promised to try every bug dish set in front of us, I would take her to the one place in Thailand she truly wanted to see: the Unicorn Cafe.

Our long and circuitous path to this unicorn mecca had actually begun some 20 years earlier, when Christina and I were having a rather heated argument over a package I had just received. It went something like this:

Christina: "No, I am putting my foot down on this one. No. No. No. You are not allowed to eat them."

Me: "What do you mean? Wait—are you actually telling me what I can and cannot eat? You don't understand. How can I talk to my students about the importance of eating insects in prehistoric diets if neither they nor I have ever eaten any? And how can I ask them to try them if I haven't?" The package was from a company called Thailand Unique. It was a big deal for Christina and me for several reasons. First, it was full of edible insects—certainly novel for both of us. We were young newlyweds, learning about ourselves and each other all the time. Every time one of us pushed a limit, the other became more aware of whom they had actually married. A box of edible insects, along with all the other limits I was pushing, seemed to have struck a nerve. Second, it was the first package I had received from overseas, meaning it was relatively expensive. Being grad students, we were broke, and it wasn't cheap to buy and ship these insects.

It floored me that in order to obtain insects suitable and legal for human consumption—at least anything more substantive than a gag gift of scorpions in lollipops or chocolate-covered ants—I had to buy them from so far away. But I firmly believed in my approach to teaching, which is based on immersing students so that they use all of their senses and pushing them beyond their comfort zone, where they truly start to learn. I'd been waiting on these edible insects to launch a new lesson focused on modern issues of human diet, health, food security, and sustainability within the context of ancestral diets. I wanted to take my modern Western 20-somethings into an entirely new experience of eating bugs, called entomophagy, get them over the "yuck" factor, and then have them look at this practice in the diets of their ancestors and their contemporaries in other parts of the world. After all, how could I expect people who had never eaten insects to engage in a meaningful dialogue about it? This was my motivation, and this was what I was trying to get across to Christina.

Eventually I convinced her, succeeded with my students, and later that year even served insects at the party after I defended my dissertation.

Why bugs? For one thing, we've probably been eating them for at least seven million years. In a diet dominated by wild vegetables and fruits, insects were the earliest food our ancestors consumed that even bordered on being nutrient-dense. The consumption of insects millions of years ago has left no archaeological trace, but we base our belief that insects made up a portion of their diet on the study of a variety of primates that serve as proxy for this practice. Today, it's estimated that at least two billion people eat bugs as part of their daily fare, according to a 2013 report by the United Nations' Food and Agriculture Organization (FAO) entitled "Edible Insects: Future Prospects for Food and Feed Security." More than 1,900 species of insects have been reported as food. "Globally, the most commonly consumed insects are beetles (Coleoptera) (31 percent); caterpillars (Lepidoptera) (18 percent); and bees, wasps, and ants (Hymenoptera) (14 percent). Following these are grasshoppers, locusts, and crickets (Orthoptera) (13 percent); cicadas, leafhoppers, planthoppers, scale insects, and true bugs (Hemiptera) (10 percent); termites (Isoptera) (3 percent); dragonflies (Odonata) (3 percent); flies (Diptera) (2 percent); and other orders (5 percent)."

The report goes on to note that while insects are a common food source around the world, in most Western countries "people view entomophagy with disgust and associate eating insects with primitive behavior" (what I call the yuck factor). "This attitude," the report says, "has resulted in the neglect of insects in agricultural research. Despite historical references to the use of insects for food, the topic of entomophagy has only very recently started to capture public attention worldwide." In order to feed the world's projected nine billion people by 2050, food production must double, the report states, stressing that land, water, and oceanic resources are limited and that we must find ways to grow food that are more sustainable and efficient to meet these needs. Insects are a logical choice. They require far fewer resources to grow than foods like beef, pork, and poultry, and pound for pound they punch far above their weight when it comes to delivering protein, vitamins, and minerals. The report notes that the "composition of unsaturated omega-3 and -6 fatty acids in mealworms is comparable with that in fish (and higher than in cattle and pigs), and the protein, vitamin, and mineral content of mealworms is similar to that in fish and meat."

While our ancestors' bug gourmet was probably akin to a primate slurping ants off a stick that's just been pulled from an ant mound, today's technologies let us consume insects in myriad ways, and it's well worth it. The same FAO report notes that 100 grams of mealworms have 20 grams of protein and 13 grams of fat; ant eggs have 14 grams of protein and 4 grams of fat; and grasshoppers have a whopping 30 grams of protein and 3.8 grams of fat. Compare that to the same quantity of 85 percent lean ground beef, which has 26 grams of protein and 15.41 grams of fat (according to the USDA FoodData Central), or two eggs, which have 12 grams of protein and 10 grams of fat.

Entomo Farms in Ontario, Canada, which specializes in crickets as the basis of their flour and powder, has also spearheaded research into crickets and mealworms as a sustainable, healthy protein source. According to their research, 100 grams of cricket flour contains 65 grams of protein, while 113 grams of beef contains just 32 grams of protein. Cricket flour includes all nine essential amino acids, has more calcium than milk, and has more iron than spinach. Entomo Farms' cricket powder contains 30 times more vitamin B_{12} than beef pound for pound, and also possesses a more ideal omega-6:omega-3 ratio of 3:1, compared to grain-fed beef — what you typically find at the grocery store — at 20:1. (Grass-fed beef is more in line with crickets, at about 3:1.) Omega-6 and omega-3, essential fatty acids that our bodies do not make on their own, help promote immune system health and lower the risk of heart disease, among other benefits. Researchers believe that our ancestors consumed a diet with an omega-6:omega-3 ratio of 1:1, and health experts today advise eating a diet with a ratio of no greater than 4:1. However, the typical Western diet has a ratio of somewhere between 15:1 and 16.7:1, and experts believe that these imbalanced proportions contribute to health issues, including cardiovascular disease, cancer, and inflammatory and autoimmune diseases.

Beyond human health, the planet's health can also benefit from a bug-based diet. According to the FAO report, insects "emit considerably fewer greenhouse gases than most livestock (methane, for instance, is produced by only a few insect groups, such as termites and cockroaches)." Likewise, ammonia emissions associated with livestock aren't a factor in insect rearing. Insects can be raised almost anywhere, so production doesn't require ownership of large tracts of land, let alone clearing of land, nor does it require massive water resources. It takes 7.5 gallons of fresh water to produce 10 grams of cricket-based protein, while the same amount of poultry protein requires 52.5 gallons of water, and beef protein 97.5 gallons.

Entomo Farms' co-founder Jarrod Goldin estimates that if a family of four eats food made from insect protein rather than red meat one day of the week, that family would save 171,712 gallons of fresh water a year. The FAO report also notes that insects, by nature of their physiology, are far better at converting feed to protein, which means it takes a whole lot less feed to produce equivalent amounts of protein from insects. "Crickets, for example, need 12 times less feed than cattle, four times less feed than sheep, and half as much feed as pigs and broiler chickens to produce the same amount of protein," the report notes.

For these and many other reasons, I have made entomophagy part of my curriculum at Washington College. I even tried to bring the concept to a larger audience by hosting insect bake sales at the college, yet even there I ran smack into Western biases. For years our bake sales were stuck beneath the steps leading up to the dining hall. We could not get permission to serve insects in the dining hall for fear that it would compromise the commercial kitchen status of the college's food facility. Every year I would call the Kent County Health Department and try to get permission, and every year they would tell me that as long as it was for a closed audience, no money changed hands, and we were not in the college's "real" cooking or dining facilities, I could do it. Think about the message this sent to our students: Insects — food that has been in our diet for millions of years and is still regularly consumed by billions of people in a variety of cultures worldwide—weren't "real" food, since they weren't allowed to be served where the "real" food was prepared and offered to students.

Finally, after something like eight years of this, we had a breakthrough. The county's food safety inspector started asking questions at the federal level about whether or not insects can be prepared in commercial kitchens and served in licensed dining facilities. Because of the odd nature of the inquiry it took some doing, but eventually she learned that insects fall under the federal Food and Drug Administration's GRAS classification— Generally Recognized as Safe. Just like salt and pepper, we could serve insects in the dining hall.

So, with an army of amazing students and staff at the college, we built a makeshift "food truck" out of cardboard, created Oaxacan-style tacos entirely from scratch (albeit using crickets rather than chapulines—grasshoppers), and served them in the dining hall. We invited Pat Crowley from Chapul, a company that makes protein bars from cricket flour, to speak to the students and help them make their own cricket flour protein bars from scratch. The next year the event was bigger. We actually took over one of the food stations in the dining hall and made insect tacos as a dinner option. We organized a series of events, including screening two documentaries on entomophagy—*Bugs: A Gastronomic Adventure with the Nordic Food Lab* and *Bugs on the Menu*. The whole thing drew enough attention that WBAL, a television station in Baltimore, asked me to do a live show about making and eating cricket tacos.

All seemed to be perfect: I was broadening the concept of entomophagy for my students in the context of their education about ancient peoples and foodways. I had read everything I could find about entomophagy, viewed everything I could on the internet, and even experimented on my own. But something was still missing, and that was context. To make insects a real part of our diet again, and to present this concept in a way that would be attractive and palatable to our bug-phobic American culture, I needed to experience cultures and people who still today routinely eat bugs. Where better to find this than where my very first foray into entomophagy began? Through a restaurant in Bangkok called Insects in the Backyard that my son Billy researched online, I connected with the

Asian Food and Feed Insect Association (AFFIA), which organized an agenda for us and set up all the contacts, a translator, meetings, and reservations. We were off to Thailand.

Our entomophagy adventure began—after my obligatory trip to the Unicorn Cafe with Alyssa—at Chef Mai Thitiwat's restaurant, Insects in the Backyard, where we got our first taste of modern cuisine fused with a Stone Age diet in a meal focused on insects. We joined Nathan Preteseille, the coordinator of the AFFIA and an innovator in insect product development, at Chef Mai's restaurant inside the Chang Chui Bangkok Plane Night Market. The meal featured several different varieties of crickets, bamboo worms, silkworm pupae, ants, and ant larvae. Entrees included nachos with silkworm cherry tomato salsa, crab and giant water beetle ravioli, lobster and grasshopper bisque risotto, pan-fried chicken breast with Japanese sweet potatoes and white crickets, fresh house-made cricket pasta with black basil pesto and chorizo, and classic Italian tiramisu made with silkworm powder.

Chef Mai did not attempt to hide the insects in the food; on the contrary, he celebrated them, offering a culinary and visual presentation of insects as food. He showed what is possible when you transform the nutrient-dense food of our ancestors in ways that meet the expectations of the modern Western palate. This approach is critical, because it's not enough to just believe in the nutrient density of the food. Biologically that makes sense, yes, but culturally we have needs that require a more calculated approach. Chef Mai was able to create dishes that surpassed what I thought could be done with bugs in terms of flavor, texture, and presentation.

The next morning, we woke early—or at least early for jet-lagged us—and scrambled downstairs to meet the taxi that would take us to the next stop on our agenda: the Khlong Toei Market. Here, Massimo Reverberi and David Pattison of Bugsolutely were to take us on a tour, focusing on edible insects for sale. We would then return to Massimo's house and the headquarters of Bugsolutely to sample his company's cricket pasta and talk about his approach to entomophagy.

The market was sensory overload. We passed live chickens in woven basket cages right next to their butchered brethren cut in half on cutting boards and displaying golden orange orbs—their unlaid eggs, a nutrient-dense delicacy—intact. We passed fish slithering across tables and jumping out of buckets. We passed mesh bags full of live bullfrogs that the vendors were happy to kill and clean for you on the spot. We saw countless pigs and cows in various states of butchering and corresponding buckets full of offal—from hearts to intestines—all for sale. Nothing went to waste.

I found something beautiful and visceral about the entire thing. There was no question where the food was coming from and who grew it, raised it, and harvested it. During every transaction, the producer and consumer interacted, a profoundly important connection that our culture has largely lost. Much of what you buy here is alive and killed in front of you. There's no doubt about the freshness. The producers get the chance to see their consumers and the families they will be feeding, and there's an inherent sense of responsibility that is absent in our own anonymous and disconnected industrialized food system.

But we were there to see the bugs! After weaving through what seemed like endless aisles of different foods, we came to the section where insects were for sale. There were four different types of crickets, grasshoppers, bamboo worms, silkworm pupae (they came from China and are a byproduct of the silk industry), water beetles, and mounds of weaver ant eggs. Even though I don't speak Thai, it was obvious that those purchasing insects weren't doing it for "survival" or because they couldn't afford anything else. In fact, many of them came to the insect stalls with bags overflowing with other food they had purchased. They were buying insects because many of them grew up eating insects. It's a traditional food source for them, complete with all of the memories associated with a food that's ingrained in a culture, just like the pumpkins and apples that Americans buy at Thanksgiving to bake pies. When we were finished, we returned to Bugsolutely, where we enjoyed a delicious meal of cricket pasta with pesto. Unlike Chef Mai, who makes insects the focal point of a dish, Massimo believes he can reach a broader population—especially Westerners—more quickly and effectively by using cricket flour to enhance the nutrition of foods we're already comfortable with. In his approach to entomophagy, he's not trying to hide the fact that there are crickets in the pasta, but he believes that putting bugs directly in someone's face will provoke the yuck factor. Instead of seeing insects as a nutrient-dense and sustainable food, people will see them as exotic pawns in a game of dare. He's certain that his product and method will make good nutrition more accessible to more people.

Our final stop in Thailand was the one about which I was most excited, a chance for me and my family to experience the culture surrounding traditional entomophagy that is typically not seen by outsiders. I wanted us to participate in the harvesting, cooking, and consumption of insects with people for whom entomophagy is a regular part of their lives. After a 40-minute flight from Bangkok to Phitsanulok, we drove an hour to the Boonchoo Weaver Ant Egg Farm. As we turned off the dirt road and headed up a lane, the jungle became dominated by mango trees that seemed to be connected by thin pieces of red twine in geometric patterns. I had no idea what I was looking at.

Boonchoo Kitsantria, the ant egg farmer, was a thin, sinewy man wearing a long-sleeved shirt, long pants, and tall rubber boots, which seemed odd in the sweltering heat. Once a mango farmer, Boonchoo realized that the eggs of the weaver ants that inhabit the mango trees would be a more productive crop than the fruit. Ant eggs have always been a traditional part of his village's diet, so it was an easy and logical switch to make. He wasted no time in enlisting our help, handing us equipment ranging from a bottle of Hale's Bluboy (a sweet red syrup), a bottle of M-150 (an energy drink similar to Red Bull), a plate with bits of leftover cooked fish and rice, a long bamboo pole with a large bag on the end, and a large dish. We followed him into the mango grove, where he stopped at a pole with a plastic crate on top.

Weaver ants weave intricate homes out of mango tree leaves, where they lay copious amounts of eggs. Boonchoo's job is to ensure the ants are well fed so that they produce as many eggs as possible, and then to harvest the eggs when the time is right. Between clumps of trees he had placed posts topped with plastic crates, in which he deposited leftovers from the previous night's meal—they could be rice, fish, rat, frog, or any combination. The baffling red lines of twine were basically ant roadways extending from the mango trees to these feeding stations. The ants could easily navigate these lines, collect the food, and return it to the queens, who lay the eggs. Hundreds and hundreds of ants swarmed the lines, lugging outsized chunks of food and sometimes working together to transport the largest pieces. The red lines also extended to bottles attached to the posts' sides and filled with sugar-rich red liquid. Each held a stick that acted as a ladder for the ants to easily climb down to drink. We mixed up a sugary Hale's Bluboy with M-150 and filled the bottles. Boonchoo included the M-150, he said, to make the ants "extra active."

Once we finished feeding the ants, Boonchoo handed me the large dish and grabbed the long pole with the bag on the end, and we walked deeper into the mango grove. He reached his pole up into a tree and used it to whack the ants and eggs from the nest. Most of them fell into the bag below, but we quickly comprehended his clothing choices; the ants that missed the bag and fell onto the ground were extremely agitated. Weaver ants are known for a fiercely painful bite, and within seconds we were all feeling it. It must have been a comical sight — Boonchoo busy harvesting ant eggs from the mango tree with his pole and bag, while a family of Americans in short pants and short-sleeved shirts danced around yelping and frantically slapping themselves to brush off angry ants! Finally, he dumped a bag full of ants and eggs into the large dish and used the breeze to winnow, casting the ants aside and leaving only the smaller, denser eggs.

After the quick harvest, Boonchoo walked us to the patio behind his house, where dishes of vegetables, fruits, rice, leaves, and weaver ant eggs waited for us to learn how to transform them into a meal. The village women showed us how to prepare ant egg salad, or yam kai mot daeng, and ant egg omelets, just like an ordinary omelet but filled with ant eggs. We learned how to fold betel leaves around the salad to use as both an edible utensil and bowl. The bitter flavors of the leaf exploded in my mouth just as the flavors of the salad did. We also enjoyed roasted crickets and a variety of fruits including mangoes, rose apples, and bananas. And, for dessert, steamed sticky rice cakes with bananas wrapped in banana leaves.

Our entomophagy adventures in Thailand were exactly what I had hoped for. It wasn't just about eating insects; I'd been doing that for years. I was seeking ways to make this nutrient-dense, sustainable food, which our ancestors and people all over the world have relied upon, acceptable and relevant in the contemporary Western diet. My family—at that time an adult woman, a high-school girl, a middle-school boy, and an elementary-school girl—was a built-in sounding board providing invaluable perspectives in understanding how to do this.

Which brings us to Alyssa, my youngest and pickiest eater. At first, it seemed that the Unicorn Cafe bribery wasn't enough. She wouldn't touch the beautifully plated dishes at Insects in the Backyard. She did a little better with Massimo's cricket pasta, but even then ate one only piece. She simply would not eat the bugs—as a food, they were too foreign and strange to her. That is, until we walked through Boonchoo's mango grove, feeding ants and enduring their irritated bites, then harvested their eggs and helped the villagers prepare the meal. Finally the barriers that the modern Western food culture and lifestyle have created for Alyssa came down. She ate the ant egg omelet, she ate the ant egg salad, and she ate the crickets.

She is not alone. Although our Western notions of food still largely resist it, entomophagy is gaining momentum and attention and finding its way into health food stores, restaurants, and other outlets. Several US cities have at least one restaurant that serves insects in some form, such as Bug Appétit in New Orleans, whose chefs cook with waxworms, mealworms, and crickets and offer dishes including cricket king cake during Mardi Gras and "chocolate chirp" cookies, on top of which a cricket takes the place of chocolate; La Condesa in Austin, whose menu includes chapulines (Oaxacan grasshoppers); Don Bugito in San Francisco, which offers insect-based snacks like dark chocolate crickets and spicy mealworms; and the Black Ant in New York City, where you can order manchego grasshopper croquettes, black ant guacamole, grasshopper tacos, and a margarita with a glass rimmed in black ant salt.

Over the past decade, businesses have sprung up to offer insect-based products that are sold in health food and specialty stores and online, such as Pat Crowley's Chapul Cricket Protein Bars and Laura D'Asaro and Rose

Wang's Chirps Chips, a line of high-protein snack chips made with cricket powder (it is interesting to note that both of these companies received investments from Mark Cuban through *Shark Tank*). In Portland, Oregon, Charles Wilson founded Cricket Flours in part to find protein and wheat alternatives to deal with food allergies, and he now sells a range of products including cricket brownie mix and roasted crickets, as well as cricket flour. Entomo Farms in Canada farms crickets on approximately 60,000 square feet, while in the US, Cowboy Cricket Farms in Montana, founded in 2016, is now expanding into a 10,000-square-foot facility. Combined with its farming partners, the new addition totals about 20,000 square feet of cricket farming.

According to a regularly updated list kept by Anders Engström on a site called Bugburger, there are at least two dozen businesses active in the US making insect-based snacks, flours, and protein powders, and more than 140 worldwide, from New Zealand to Finland and Israel to the Netherlands. In a major step toward the approval of snacks and other foods that contain insects in the European Union, the European Food Safety Authority in late 2020 ruled that dried yellow mealworms, in whole and powdered form, are safe for human consumption. A *Bloomberg Green* report on the decision noted that the global insect farming business is attracting financing from businesses like Cargill and Nestlé, and the Singapore-based market research firm Arcluster predicted that by 2025 it will exceed $4.1 billion. The market research company Global Market Insights, in a February 2020 "Edible Insect Market Analysis," noted that the global market size for edible insects was at $112 million in 2019 and projected to expand at a compound annual growth rate of 47 percent, to $1.5 billion, between 2019 and 2026. In a release announcing the report, the firm said that insect-based protein bars would command a large market and noted that a demand for high-protein, economical food sources and "shifting trends in dietary needs" would propel growth. Yet another industry analyst, IndustryARC, in a report on the insect protein market between 2021 and 2026, estimated global market revenues at $62.5 million in 2018, with a projected compound annual growth rate of 21 percent from 2019 to 2025.

All of this bodes well for making it easier for people to get past the yuck factor and incorporate insect protein into their diets. Although there is still some difficulty in obtaining fresh insects and certain specialties such as ant eggs and cockroaches (even though it's simple to order chapulines online), it's easy to work with insect proteins in your kitchen. Cricket and other insect powders are easily purchased online and in health food stores and can be added to practically anything—smoothies, yogurt, baked goods (by substituting up to 20 percent of the flour), dressings, sauces, and even coffee—to enhance the nutritional content of the food. This addition increases important proteins, fats, and minerals without negatively impacting the texture, flavor, or color of the final product. That said, be careful if you have a shellfish allergy; insect and crustacean exoskeletons are very similar, so if you have a shellfish allergy, you may also be allergic to insects. Adding insect powders to foods is certainly a sustainable way to boost nutritional value in your diet. For the more adventurous cooks, I have included a few insect recipes that are designed for easily accessible dry-roasted crickets and cricket flour.

TIPS AND RECIPES

INCORPORATING INSECT FLOURS IN YOUR BAKING

An easy and accessible way to incorporate insects in your diet is to substitute up to 20 percent cricket flour for wheat or other grain flour in recipes. This will increase important proteins, fats, and minerals without negatively impacting the texture, flavor, or color of the final product.

CRICKET POWER BALLS

Most protein and power bars are filled with artificial sweeteners, sugar alcohols, and food industry byproducts passed off as nutritional additives or contain so much sugar they should be considered candy bars. Convenient, yes. Healthy, no. These cricket power balls take only a few minutes to make, store well, and are convenient on-the-go food you can feel good about feeding your family. They rely on sustainable and nourishing insects for their protein, use coconut oil for their fat, and are minimally sweetened with the perfect amounts of dates and raw honey to draw out the flavor from the cocoa powder.

1 cup sunflower seed flour

1 cup unsweetened shredded coconut, plus extra for rolling

⅔ cup high-quality cocoa powder

½ cup organic cricket flour

⅓ cup virgin coconut oil

¼ cup raw honey

16 regular or 8 Medjool pitted dates

Combine all the ingredients in a food processor and process until smooth. Divide the mixture into 20 equal portions and roll into balls with your hands until uniform, then roll in additional shredded coconut to coat. Cover and store at room temperature for several days, in the refrigerator for several weeks, or in the freezer for several months.

CRICKET GRANOLA

This granola is unlike any you have ever made or tried. The oats and seeds are rendered as safe and nourishing as possible by soaking them overnight (the oats in fermented dairy such as yogurt or kefir, and the seeds in salted water). The nutritional content skyrockets above traditional granola thanks to the addition of the yogurt and crickets. And, although they are still visible, the shape and crunch of the crickets are right at home among the rest of the ingredients. This is a nut- and fruit-free granola, but feel free to add whatever nuts or dried fruit you like.

2 cups rolled oats
¾ cup plain yogurt or Kefir (page 181)
⅓ cup sunflower seeds
⅓ cup pumpkin seeds
1 tablespoon plus pinch sea salt, divided
2 tablespoons coconut oil, plus more for greasing
1 cup shredded coconut
¾ cup roasted crickets
3 tablespoons raw honey
3 tablespoons pure maple syrup
½ teaspoon pure vanilla extract
¼ teaspoon ground cinnamon

Soak the oats: Combine the rolled oats and fermented dairy (yogurt or kefir) in a medium bowl. Mix thoroughly, cover, and allow to soak and ferment overnight on the counter.

Soak the seeds: Combine the sunflower and pumpkin seeds in a medium bowl. Cover with about 1 inch of warm water and add 1 tablespoon sea salt. Stir to dissolve the salt, then cover and leave overnight on the counter. The next morning drain, rinse well, and drain again.

Preheat the oven to 300°F. Grease a rimmed baking sheet with coconut oil.

Combine the oat-yogurt mixture, drained seeds, shredded coconut, crickets, and coconut oil in a large bowl. Using clean hands, incorporate the coconut oil until it's evenly distributed. The heat of your hands will gently melt the coconut oil and allow it to coat the ingredients. In a separate bowl, whisk together the honey, maple syrup, vanilla, cinnamon, and a pinch of salt. Combine with the granola and mix well with a spoon. Distribute the granola evenly on the prepared baking sheet. Bake, stirring occasionally, for 1 hour, or until browned.

Let the granola cool, then store it in an airtight container at room temperature for several months.

CHILI-LIME CRICKETS

These crickets are made in the Oaxacan tradition of chapulines, the fried grasshoppers coated with chili powder and sprinkled with lime juice that are sold by vendors in the large open markets and on the street. These are incredibly versatile and can be eaten as is for a snack, sprinkled on top of guacamole, or included in salsa. But my favorite way to eat them is to wrap them in a nixtamalized Tortilla (page 160) and add minced onion, Crema (page 187), and fresh cilantro for a delicious and nourishing taco.

> 1 tablespoon lard, tallow, or butter
> 1 cup roasted crickets
> Juice and grated zest of 1 lime
> ½ teaspoon chili powder
> Sea salt

Heat the fat in a large skillet over medium heat. Add the crickets and lime juice and stir until the lime juice has been absorbed and the crickets are warmed through. Add the chili powder and salt to taste and stir until evenly distributed. Transfer to a bowl, top with the lime zest, and serve.

CRICKET RILLETTES

MAKES 3 (4-OUNCE) RAMEKINS

Rillettes, a form of potted meat, are a great way to use leftover meat scraps and introduce a whole new level of flavor and nutrition by adding bone broth and rich animal fat. The entire thing is topped with a layer of melted fat, creating an airtight seal that increases shelf life. In this recipe, the meat is replaced with roasted crickets and rehydrated with broth before combining with fat. The bone broth and fat can come from any animal or, for those of you who want to introduce insects into your diet but wish to stay away from other animal foods, the combination of vegetable broth and coconut oil works just fine. This makes a great spread for Butter Bite Crackers (page 133).

4 thyme sprigs
1 rosemary sprig
3 whole black peppercorns
1 cup roasted crickets
1 cup Trash Bone Broth (page 79) or vegetable broth
¾ cup lard, butter, tallow, bacon grease, or coconut oil
Pinch sea salt

Make a sachet by placing the thyme, rosemary, and peppercorns in a small piece of cloth (cheesecloth works great). Gather the sides and tie them together with a piece of string to create a small bag. Combine the crickets, broth, and sachet in a small saucepan. Bring to a boil over medium heat. As soon as the mixture reaches a boil, turn off the heat and cover for 15 minutes to let the crickets absorb the broth and rehydrate.

In a small saucepan, melt the fat over low heat.

Drain the crickets in a colander and discard the sachet. Transfer the rehydrated crickets to a blender or food processor, add ½ cup of the melted fat and the salt, and pulse to break up and blend until smooth.

Tightly pack the cricket mixture into three ramekins or small mason jars and cap with a layer of the remaining melted fat.

Let cool completely. The rillettes can be stored, covered, in the refrigerator for up to 1 week or in the freezer for several months. Allow to come to room temperature before serving.

Chapter 8

EARTH, ASH, AND CHARCOAL

HAVE YOUR FIRE AND EAT IT, TOO

Hanging on for dear life inside the passenger van, I tried not to look out the window. I wasn't sweating just from the heat as we bumped and churned down the side of a mountain in the northern Rift Valley of Kenya. There wasn't much left of this road after recent rains had washed most of it off the mountain. Guardrails? What were they? Every time I risked looking over my shoulder, I had a heart-stopping view of the sheer drop of several thousand feet we'd hurtle down if our driver made one wrong move or the road just evaporated. I've asked my family to travel all over the world with me to see and experience firsthand how traditional cultures approach food, health, sustainability, and diet, but I was seriously wondering whether I'd gone too far this time. It had seemed like a great idea when our guide, Samuel, assured us that if we traveled deeper into the lowlands of West Pokot, we'd find people who still produced and consumed the fabled ash yogurt—known as mursik—as part of their daily diets. Once nomadic pastoralists, the Pokot people could easily produce and transport mursik as a staple food for herders while they were grazing their livestock. Today, these people generally live in permanent villages, but they continue to raise goats and cows whose milk they use for this traditional yogurt. Some believe it is so beneficial to health that it's one reason Kenya produces some of the world's most powerful runners and athletes. In fact, in some parts of Kenya, when athletes return home from winning races around the world, they're feted with a celebration that includes a ceremonial drink of mursik. I couldn't pass up a chance to learn more about a food this ancient and fascinating, although I was having my doubts until finally, after almost three hours of tense travel down the mountains, we reached the lowlands and the road flattened out. It wasn't much better, but at least we weren't on the verge of plunging to our deaths anymore, just maybe being jostled into jelly. Eventually, we turned off the road and drove into the bush, stopping at the entrance to a village of round wattle-and-daub huts with thatched roofs.

We heard them from a distance before we saw them, the sound of singing, bells, and then the people in their bright clothing, dancing toward us. They surrounded us in a sea of color and music, and invited us to dance with them through the gate into the village. Eventually they showed us into one of the homes, where we sat on the hard-packed dirt floor and watched as three women huddled around a small fire burning in the hearth. The critical tools for this process were a long-necked gourd like a calabash, decorated with cowrie shells, and a thick, rough stick, which we learned was wood from a tree known locally as a kromwo, *Ozoroa insignis*. One of the women stuck an end of the stick into the fire until it was glowing red. Then, gripping the stick with a gnarled fist, she pushed it into the gourd and vigorously scraped it up and down along the gourd's insides. Smoke billowed from the mouth of the gourd as she scraped, and she continued to repeat this process—heating the stick red hot, then scraping and pushing—until the entire inside of the gourd was scoured and coated with fine, black charcoal. She also used the red-hot stick to wipe and scrape the inside of a small lid made from the cut-off end of the gourd. She shook out the gourd, scattering bits of excess charcoal on the floor. Then she filled it with raw cow's milk, which quickly turned from white to a speckled blue-gray. After she capped the gourd, it would be set aside to ferment for up to three months, but typically at three days, it's ready to drink. The women explained that it can also ferment for over six months while it loses moisture and becomes more like cheese than yogurt. In this case, it becomes what is called *cheposoyo*, and during times of hunger, a spoonful mixed with water a few times a day is sometimes the only food available. The women offered us several-months-old mursik made from raw goat's milk, and its complex flavor was remarkable. The kids went back for seconds of this nourishing food that was made of nothing more than raw milk and wood ash.

We would witness this process twice while in Kenya. And, as with drinking blood and milk with the Samburu, the experience gets to the core of something we've been bumping into obliquely all along: What is considered "normal" food? We have already covered foods the Western food system considers "fringe," like wild greens, offal, and raw milk, in the context of ancient and traditional processing technologies. We have seen how their nutrition can be incorporated into our contemporary diets, much to our benefit not only in terms of health but also in reestablishing more direct connections to our food. Rather than banning certain foods from our tables, we have learned that by asking "*How* should I eat this?" we can change our perceptions while applying techniques that have proven their worth and ingenuity through the ages. Why not take it a step further and explore the boundaries of what seems to constitute food itself?

For example, ash and charcoal. These are often used interchangeably, but they have distinct qualities and benefits. Ash is what is left over after a fire has completely burned in the presence of oxygen, and charcoal is what remains when something organic is subjected to high heat in the absence of oxygen. Ash is typically gray, fragile, light, and feathery, while charcoal is black and gritty. (Interestingly, while the mursik we had in Kenya is known as ash yogurt, it's technically charcoal that is coating the end of the superheated stick.) Historically, ash was used as a chemical leavening agent in baking. In fact, the baking soda you undoubtedly have in your pantry can trace its roots directly to ash. It was invented as a replacement for ash and ash-derived products such as potash. Colonial American homes would have an ash hopper outside where ashes from the hearth were placed and rain could seep through them. After the lye-rich water beneath was collected and boiled, potash remained. Baking potash in a kiln burned off the carbon impurities and resulted in the more refined pearlash. According to SmithsonianMag.com, pearlash is mentioned in *American Cookery,* the first American cookbook, published in 1796. In 1846, bicarbonate of soda, aka baking soda, was first manufactured in the US; when mixed with an acid like buttermilk, baking soda also reacts to produce carbon dioxide. (This was still a labor-intensive solution, and eventually chemists took this culinary conundrum one step further by inventing baking powder. Baking powder includes tartaric acid—a winemaking byproduct—which provides the acid needed for the chemical reaction and doesn't require mixing together two somewhat tricky agents to achieve the desired effect.)

But we were adding ash to our foods long before our Colonial forebears were wrestling with how to get their biscuits to rise. We've seen that for thousands of years Mesoamericans mixed ash with water to nixtamalize their maize. And anyone who's cooked over an open fire can easily imagine how our ancestors would have been getting ash in their foods. Even the slightest of breezes effortlessly dislodges the feathery ash from the fire, and when it takes flight, it seems to coat everything from steaks grilling over coals to marshmallows toasting on the end of a stick. Evidence in the archaeological record indicates that early humans used wood ash; a find in Qesem Cave in Israel dating from 300,000 years ago reveals that our ancestors treated deer legs with ash, most likely as a preservative. Among other examples are Roman gladiators who drank a tonic of ashes after training and the Yanomami of Brazil and Venezuela, who would consume ashes of deceased humans as part of a cannibalism ritual.

Ash's alkaline characteristics can alter the environment within which food is processed. producing a multitude of benefits. A source of essential minerals such as calcium, manganese, iron, copper, zinc, sodium, magnesium, potassium, and phosphorus, ash acts to detoxify and restore balance in our bodies, its alkaline base counteracting the acids we take in from our environment. Today, ash is a component in some of the world's best cheeses, including the French Morbier and the Californian Humboldt Fog, because it changes the microenvironment in and around the cheese, producing desirable effects. For instance, as cheese ages, it continues to slowly ferment, increasing acidity. In some cheese this acidity inhibits ripening. Ash neutralizes the acidity and helps promote certain ripening processes. Also, the environment produced by coating a cheese with ash attracts certain favorable molds, such as *Penicillium candidum,* which is essential to the production of the white mold that coats cheeses like Brie and Camembert.

In some cheeses that required more than a day's worth of milk to create, such as Morbier, ash was used to keep the flies off the cheese until the next day's curd was added; today that tradition is carried forward, although more for aesthetics and flavor than to repel bugs. Aesthetically, using ash as part of the process can result in a cheese that is complex and even beautiful when presented on the plate. The thin, smoky line of ash bisecting the creamy cheese in Humboldt Fog conjures a layer of the eponymous mist hovering over the bay.

Charcoal is an even more powerful natural detoxifier than ash. In its approved medicinal form, activated charcoal is a fine powder produced from superheating materials rich in carbon like wood and peat to enhance and maximize its ability to adsorb — or chemically bond with — certain molecules. As such, it's frequently used as an emergency treatment for drug overdoses or poisoning; the activated charcoal bonds with the toxins, and because the human body doesn't absorb charcoal, the combined material passes safely through and out of the digestive tract. Activated charcoal is also used in everyday items like in-home water filters, in which it adsorbs certain chemicals, like chlorine, while leaving others, like sodium, alone. While activated charcoal is a separately produced substance, the ability of ordinary charcoal to bond with toxins can still be beneficial. (The difference between charcoal and activated charcoal is that activated charcoal has been treated in ways that force its pores to open up, increase the surface area, and become more adsorbent.)

It is difficult to determine whether charcoal found in the archaeological record was consumed. However, we know that our ancestors had access to charcoal as far back as two million years ago, when they first controlled fire; and since fire was the heat source for cooking, charcoal was always around food. We know that charcoal was used in creating black color in cave art for tens of thousands of years. It was used as a binder in different glues and mastics for attaching two different things to one another, like an arrowhead to a shaft or a stone knife blade to a handle. It was essential to providing the continuous high heat necessary during the Bronze Age to purify metals and create alloys. During the Iron Age, it provided the carbon required to turn iron into steel. Along with saltpeter and sulfur, it's an essential component of gunpowder, which was invented in the ninth century.

Consuming charcoal does not increase our nutrient intake, but it can physically trap certain toxins and prevent our bodies from assimilating them, and its medicinal values have been documented on papyrus since as early as 1500 BC. Physically, charcoal is incredibly porous, since the intense heat needed to make it eliminates everything but the carbon. This provides enormous area to adsorb toxins (though not all toxins; for example, it's ineffective against cyanide, alcohol, metals, and strong acids and bases). Some consider it the most powerful antidote known to humans, and its proponents have gone to extreme measures to prove it. In the 19th century, French chemist Michel Bertrand survived after swallowing a lethal dose of arsenic mixed with charcoal; and in 1830, French pharmacists swallowed 10 lethal doses of strychnine with an equal amount of charcoal in front of the French Academy of Medicine.

More recently, it's become fashionable for chefs to include charcoal in their dishes. In 2018, this new trend culminated in the first-ever charcoal food festival, "50 Shades of Charcoal," where more than 15 chefs gathered in San Francisco to share their trendiest drinks and foods containing charcoal. However, despite its presence in our ancestral and traditional diets, medicinal benefits, and growing popularity, charcoal has been banned from food served in New York City restaurants. And while it remains perfectly legal in Europe, Australia, and New Zealand, it's not on the US Food and Drug Administration's Generally Regarded as Safe (GRAS) list. For this reason, chefs and others producing food commercially are restricted from using charcoal as an ingredient in the US. However, you can legally purchase food-grade charcoal online and use it in your own kitchen. When I consider the fact that a substance like corn syrup is perfectly acceptable while charcoal is not, I can only believe these sorts of rules are the result of lack of knowledge and understanding rather than factual science.

Ash and charcoal are substances our forebears were constantly coming into contact with. They weren't alien; they were part of daily life. So using them in our cooking isn't such a stretch. But what about earth? It is hard for us today to even think about the possible benefits of a diet that includes earth. We live in a culture that instantly equates dirt and soil with being dirty or soiled. While we know most of the plants we eat grow in soil (hydroponic gardens being a notable exception), we don't want to see it, let alone consume it. The veggies in our grocery stores are perfectly, unnaturally clean. If we do bring home fresh vegetables from the local farmer's market, we make sure to scrub off any dirt still clinging to the roots. In fact, our Western culture deems geophagy — the eating of earth — a form of illness, called pica. The American Psychological Association defines pica as "a rare eating disorder marked by a persistent craving for unnatural, nonnutritive substances, such as plaster, paint, hair, starch, or dirt." However, dirt — including earth and clay — does have nutritive properties, and geophagy has been practiced around the world for millennia. While in some eras and cultures it has been treated with suspicion and even derision, in others consuming earth or clay is a common and accepted practice for detoxifying foods and easing a variety of ills often related to digestion and pregnancy, and providing much-needed minerals in times of nutritional stress.

Geophagy is common throughout the animal kingdom, and it makes sense that it is a human activity as well. Evidence for geophagy in our ancestral dietary past dates to more than two million years ago at the site of Kalambo Falls in Zambia. There, according to esteemed British archaeologist J. Desmond Clark in his book *Kalambo Falls Prehistoric Site,* researchers uncovered remains of *Homo habilis,* the earliest member of our genus, *Homo,* next to a particular calcium-rich clay. The context of the discovery, in addition to the clay's suitability for detoxification, led archaeologists to believe that this early ancestor may have been using the clay as a dietary supplement. Hippocrates provided the first known written reference to geophagy in humans; he noted that pregnant women may feel "the desire to eat earth and charcoal." Pliny wrote about a kind of porridge called alica made with red clay and used to soothe ulcers "in the humid part of the body such as the mouth or anus" and as a way to stop diarrhea. In the early 1800s, German naturalist Alexander von Humboldt traveled through the Americas, and in South America he witnessed the indigenous Otomacs eating earth: "They wolf it down in quite considerable amounts." Today, in Bolivia, *p'asa* (or *phasa*) is the Aymara word for dipping native potatoes in clay as they are eaten (more on that in a bit). Archaeological evidence of this practice from Chirpa, Bolivia, dates back 2,500 years, but it's undoubtedly much older since potatoes were domesticated at least 10,000 years ago. In Sardinia, pan'ispeli (acorn bread) dates from pre-Roman times and was made with acorns from either the holm or downy oak, clay, and ash from grapevines or downy oak. In a 2012 paper, a postgraduate student at the University of Sassari in Italy documented what is still known about this bread-making, noting that the clay neutralized the tannins in the acorns and added iron and other minerals, while the ash was thought to facilitate cooking. "A further step was to strain the acorns when the mixture reached the desired consistency and quickly form little flat cakes of irregular shape. They were dried in the sun or the fireplace, in which case they were sprinkled with ashes to prevent them from sticking...It was a rustic food for men who needed energy for heavy work...The rest of the mixture was cooked until it resembled cornmeal. It was formed into many little pieces of bread... given to children, the ill, and the elderly. It was almost like a sweet and was often eaten with whey from ricotta cheese to ease digestion."

Even today, traditional societies throughout the world continue to engage in the intentional consumption of earth to supplement diets, especially during times of hunger or increased nutritional need such as pregnancy or lactation. Earth provides minerals important to our bodies such as calcium, iron, and magnesium, and it can also provide medicinal benefit, acting as an antidiarrheal and antacid. In Africa, studies have found that up to 80 percent of women consume clay, especially when they are pregnant, because it helps with morning sickness and digestion. In 2011, a Cornell University scientist researched nearly 500 accounts of geophagy worldwide. Closer to home, one of the original ingredients in Kaopectate—and where it got its name—is kaolinite, a clay mineral whose adsorbent properties act as a detoxifier. Much like charcoal, it binds to toxins and allows us to safely pass them. Kaolinite and bentonite clay continue to be consumed worldwide as digestive aids, and it's not uncommon to see chunks of them for sale in open markets in Africa and other regions.

Consuming and cooking in earth is another way in which our ancient dietary practices helped us obtain nutrition from otherwise inaccessible foods. Soil is rich with a host of probiotic cultures beneficial to the human biome. There are hundreds of different species of soil-based probiotics (SBOs), and an entire branch of the nutritional supplement industry focuses on supplying customers with them in forms called homeostatic soil organisms, bacterial soil organisms, or soil organisms. Cutting-edge chefs and food pioneers like forager Pascal Baudar are returning to cooking with earth for these reasons, as well as to harness and celebrate earth's aromas and flavors. Some fermenters also use soil-based bacteria as a medium within which to lacto-ferment vegetables. Kenyan plant expert, forager, cheesemaker, and fermenter Sue Brown ferments the soil around her home to produce a probiotic-rich drink that she consumes every day. Chef Justin Cournoyer serves a dish of radish and carrots with soil-infused butter at his restaurant Actinolite in Toronto; Chef Ben Shewry cooks potatoes in the soil in which they grew at his restaurant, Attica, in Melbourne, Australia; Chef Toshio Tanabe uses soil to create dishes from salads to gratins at his restaurant Ne Quittez Pas in Tokyo, in what he calls tsuchi ryōri, or earth cuisine; and Chef Joan Roca uses a vacuum distiller to extract the perfume of freshly dug Catalonian soil and apply it, as a foam, to an oyster dessert at his restaurant El Celler de Can Roca. In stark contrast to the fear and disdain the modern world holds for soil, these examples focus on harnessing and embracing soil as a healthy and exciting component of our diets. After all, vegetables and fruits, both staples in our diets, are essentially vehicles that we use to draw nutrients from the soil and transform them into something from which we can derive nutrition and pleasure. Geophagy, soil fermentation, and cooking in soil are all techniques to bypass that system and allow us to derive certain nutrition directly from the soil.

Potatoes are an excellent example of how the binding agents in certain clays and earth can be used to make a toxic food safe to eat. Wild potatoes and many ancient heirloom varieties have high levels of toxins such as glycoalkaloids. Even low doses of glycoalkaloids can result in abdominal pain, diarrhea, and bloating, while high doses can result in paralysis and death. In fact, all potatoes have some level of glycoalkaloids in them, even the modern varieties in our grocery stores. That's why some people have adverse reactions to eating potatoes, and why some diet gurus advocate removing potatoes from our diets. But this sort of extremism flies in the face of thousands of years of human evolution and food-processing technologies. Instead of removing entire categories of foods from our diets—whether potatoes, meat, plants, or dairy—we can rethink our approach to foods like this by connecting with the methods still used in traditional societies.

This is why I flew to Bolivia—via four different countries—enduring a terrible bout of altitude sickness when I arrived at El Alto International Airport in La Paz, at 13,000 feet the highest-altitude international airport in the world. I was bound for the Pongonhuyo-Wilajahuira community in the Andes Mountains, where I was going to live for a week with a family of indigenous Aymara Indians to learn about the different ways they detoxify native varieties of potatoes, and their practice of p'asa, dipping native potatoes in clay as they are eaten. I had read a brief account of p'asa in graduate school nearly 20 years earlier and had wanted to try it ever since. The Aymara are among the few people who still practice p'asa, and I wanted to experience it with them and learn all about the process.

After my rough start adjusting to the altitude, my guide, Catalina Huanca, and our driver took us even higher into the Altiplano, the high, treeless, rolling plains of the Andes. The city of La Paz gave way to smaller villages of brick homes and buildings, then hamlets of scattered adobe structures. We passed Lake Titicaca and eventually left the pavement for a dirt road riddled with potholes that rocked our small, two-wheel-drive vehicle from side to side like a rambunctious amusement park ride. Animals began to outnumber people, and eventually we left the road entirely, the native grasses swatting the sides of the car, until we dropped into a dried riverbed, jostling and navigating through rocks and ruts. We finally arrived at the home of Catalina's parents, Juana and Francisco, where I spent several days stumbling along with my very slow Spanish (Juana and Francisco spoke primarily Aymara, so speaking Spanish slowly was actually helpful for our communications) and learning almost more than I could take in.

The first thing Francisco showed me was how to build a hornito, a small earthen oven typical of the Camacho province where he is from. After excavating a shallow pit, he used chunks of earth to create a dome over the pit and then lit a fire within using grass and cow patties. We continued to fuel the fire for about an hour with dried cow patties until the oven's color had changed noticeably from gray-white to a darker brown and gray. At this point, Francisco began to methodically load in some of the wide array of heirloom potatoes he was cooking, then dismantled part of the oven on top of them. He repeated this process — adding potatoes, knocking down more of the oven — until the potatoes were fully surrounded by the hot chunks of earth. As the final step, he entirely covered the crushed earth and potatoes with finer dirt. "Cuarenta minutos," Francisco said, and had me set my iPhone timer.

After we excavated the oven, we carried the hot potatoes in baskets to the shade of an adobe shed as Catalina's sister, Carmen, and Juana arrived with three small bowls — two empty and one filled with salt. They also brought two earthenware jars, each containing a different-colored viscous liquid, one gray-white, the other a green like that of guacamole. Juana spread a sack on the ground and dumped the cooked potatoes onto it. She then smacked them with a grass whisk to let the strong afternoon Altiplano winds carry any remaining dirt away. She added salt to the empty bowls, stirred each jar, then poured their contents into the two bowls. This created waja, the clay dip, made from two different types of clay that each had its own flavor profile and characteristics.

They showed me the proper way to enjoy p'asa, starting with breaking the potatoes open to reveal the perfectly cooked white interior sparkling in the sun. Next, we dipped the potatoes in the waja, allowing the clay, water, and salt mixture to soak into the soft flesh. The clay dipping sauces were surprising in different ways. Without any grit or texture, they were as smooth as a creamy sauce you would expect at a fine restaurant. They also added a subtle flavor to the potatoes, one slightly sweet and the other slightly sour. Throughout my ethnographic research in Bolivia and then Peru, everywhere I went, people ate potatoes, and though they were prepared in a number of ways, the skin — which carries the vast majority of this food's dangerous toxins—was always removed first. This was the sole exception. We had no ill effects eating even some of the most toxic varieties with the skins on; to me, this speaks to the power of clay to detoxify food. There wasn't anything strange to me about dipping potatoes in clay; it all felt perfectly normal in the context of this family, community, and place. This clearly was a food that Catalina's family relished. In fact, when we had finished eating all of the potatoes, some waja remained in the bowls until Carmen, with a swipe of her finger, made sure to get every last bit— just as my kids do with mayonnaise!

I've always been fascinated by the seemingly strange things that people over the ages have learned to eat to extract the maximum amount of nutrition from even the most desolate of environments. Many of us wouldn't consider eating earth, ash, charcoal, or clay, and we look askance at people who continue to use these materials in their foodways as if they are primitive or strange. But, if we take an honest, self-reflective look at our own environments, who is really living with richer, more secure, and more sustainable food resources? Is it the people of West Pokot, who rely on nutrient- and probiotic-dense ash yogurt that has fermented for several months to make it through times of hunger? Is it the Aymara, who depend upon ubiquitous and diverse varieties of potatoes cooked in cow dung and earth and dipped in clay? Or is it we who live in places where, with the exception of wild plants sprouting through the sidewalk cracks, there are no remaining naturally occurring food sources, and who subsist on food that is shipped from places we've never seen, felt, or known? By opening our perceptions to broader concepts of what constitutes "normal" food, we create an opportunity to make the most of every food in every way that we can. And, we can take a new approach to addressing the critical issues of food security, safety, and health that are facing us as humans throughout the world.

TIPS AND RECIPES

SOURCING EDIBLE CLAY, ASH, AND CHARCOAL

Not all clays are created equal, and finding edible clay is more difficult than grabbing a shovel and heading into the backyard. Safely and successfully digging your own edible clay requires intimate knowledge of the land and an understanding of its clay types. Luckily, a large variety of high-quality edible clays are easily available online for purchase. Best choice? Look for montmorillonite powder (sometimes labeled as bentonite), which detoxifies and provides a host of minerals for the body.

You can purchase ash from cheesemaking suppliers, and food-grade activated charcoal is available online. Or, you can use ash or charcoal from a hardwood fire you build yourself — just be sure to never use ash or charcoal that comes from coal, conifers such as pine, spruce, or hemlock, or from wood that has been chemically treated or painted. Whether your charcoal has been activated and arrives on your doorstep in a cardboard box or is culled from your firepit out back and ground by hand, it has beneficial properties, from detoxifying to changing the color, character, and texture of your food.

CHARCOAL CRACKERS

Makes about 200 crackers

While it's true that at present, restaurants and food producers in the US are not allowed to include charcoal in their food, it continues to be used in foods produced in other countries. And it's available for purchase online so that you can make your own foods at home using this unique ingredient. These crackers are delicious, and when presented on a charcuterie board they are consistent showstoppers.

> 450 grams (2 cups) mature sourdough mother culture
>   (see page 128)
> 221 grams (1⅓ cups) whole wheat flour
> 9 grams (1½ teaspoons) sea salt
> 66 grams (⅓ cup) butter, room temperature, plus additional
>   melted butter for brushing
> 9 grams (2 teaspoons) finely ground charcoal or activated
>   charcoal
> Maldon salt

Combine the sourdough mother, flour, salt, softened butter, and charcoal in the bowl of a stand mixer fitted with the dough hook and mix on speed 1 until all the ingredients are fully incorporated. (Or, if mixing by hand, stir with a Danish dough whisk or wooden spoon to combine the ingredients until it becomes too difficult to continue. Turn out the dough onto a clean work surface and knead just until all the ingredients are fully incorporated.) Wrap the dough or place it in an airtight container and refrigerate for 6 to 12 hours to slowly ferment.

Preheat the oven to 350°F. Line several rimmed baking sheets with parchment paper.

Roll the dough into thin sheets (approximately 1/16 inch thick) with a rolling pin or pasta machine. Carefully transfer the dough sheets to the prepared baking sheets, cut into 1½-inch squares, brush the tops with melted butter, and sprinkle with Maldon salt. Bake for 20 to 25 minutes, until crisp and slightly browned. Transfer to a wire rack to cool. When completely cool, store in an airtight container at room temperature, up to several weeks.

CLAY SMOOTHIE

MAKES ABOUT 2 CUPS

There was a time when Christina and I drank this shake every day for breakfast. We loved starting the day by flooding our bodies with the probiotics found in kefir, the texture of the nut butter, and the soothing effects of the clay. Plus, we enjoyed the hint of sweetness delivered by the fruit and raw honey.

We no longer drink this every morning because we realize how much sugar is in fruit like bananas, and we don't want to consume the oxalates and antinutrients in nut butters so often. However, this recipe remains an excellent source of nutrition and flavor, and we whip up one of these shakes anytime we need a quick, nourishing snack or meal.

  1 cup Kefir (page 181), Mesophilic Yogurt (page 183),
     or Thermophilic Yogurt (page 185)
  ½ banana and/or other fresh fruit
  1 tablespoon nut or seed butter
  1 teaspoon edible clay (montmorillonite)
  1 teaspoon raw honey (optional)

Combine all the ingredients in a blender and blend on high speed until smooth.

CHARCOAL MAYONNAISE

MAKES ABOUT 1½ CUPS

The way we perceive food is influenced by a combination of factors, including flavor, aroma, satiation, context, and presentation. Adding charcoal to this already nourishing recipe creates a unique color, and this visual change impacts the overall dining experience; after all, how often do we get to eat black food? Plus, we can take advantage of charcoal's detoxification properties. This makes a fantastic dipping sauce for Lacto-Fries (page 58).

2 large egg yolks
1 garlic clove, minced (optional)
½ teaspoon Fermented Mustard (page 103) or Dijon mustard
Sea salt
1 cup avocado oil
1 teaspoon white wine vinegar, or more if needed
½ teaspoon finely ground charcoal or activated charcoal powder
Juice of ½ lemon

Set a medium bowl on top of a kitchen towel or moistened paper towel on the counter. This will help keep the bowl from moving as you whisk. Put the egg yolks, garlic (if using), mustard, and a pinch of salt in the bowl and whisk together. Gradually add about half the oil, very slowly at first, drop by drop, while whisking continuously. Once the emulsion is established, increase the flow of oil into a thin stream. After you have added about half the oil, whisk in the vinegar; this will loosen the mixture slightly, making it easier to incorporate the remainder of the oil. Continue to gradually add the remaining oil, whisking continuously. Add the charcoal powder and whisk to thoroughly distribute. Season with another pinch of salt, the lemon juice, and a little more vinegar, if needed. Store in a clean jar in the fridge for up to 1 week.

ASH SALT

MAKES ABOUT ½ CUP

Making ash salt from vegetable ends, stems, and skins is a great way to make use of leftovers and support a zero-waste approach in your kitchen. Onions, garlic, leeks, and other alliums, as well as celery and carrots, make fantastic choices. Use the ash salt whenever you want a little extra flavor and character; it is particularly good on meat and vegetables. One note: Some studies have found that grilling meat can produce a carcinogen known as polycyclic aromatic hydrocarbon, and cooking starchy foods like potatoes at high temperatures produces acrylamides, also carcinogens. However, this doesn't seem to be an issue when charring plant materials and vegetables to render charcoal or ash.

> 2 cups vegetable scraps from onions, garlic, leeks, celery, and/or carrots
> 2 tablespoons sea salt

Preheat the oven to 500°F with a rack in the top position.

Arrange the vegetable scraps in a single layer on a rimmed baking sheet. Bake for 1 to 2 hours, until the vegetables are completely charred.

Fully cool the vegetable scraps. Pulverize them in a spice grinder or blender and sift through a fine-mesh sieve. Mix with an equal volume of salt. Store in an airtight container at room temperature, up to several months.

Chapter 9

SUGAR

OR, THE BIRTHDAY CAKE DILEMMA

Brianna and I closed and relocked the iron gate, the only opening in the seven-foot-tall stone wall near our small cottage. Passing through the gate was something like opening the wardrobe to Narnia. It divided two completely different worlds: the 38-acre working farm on which my family and I lived for a year, and Dundrum, a suburb of Dublin, Ireland, only 15 minutes from the center of the city. Four train stops and 20 minutes later, we walked into the beautiful, buzzing kitchen of Kevin Thornton, a two-star Michelin chef and arguably Ireland's most famous cooking personality. With his wife, Muriel, Kevin owned Dublin's world-famous Thornton's Restaurant for 26 years, and more recently he's become known for his work on the popular TV series *Heat* and *Guerrilla Gourmet*. Now, he and Muriel have remodeled their gorgeously appointed kitchen into a teaching space called Kevin Thornton's KOOKS, where they teach master classes in an intimate setting.

We were here for a class on petit fours and macarons to celebrate Brianna's 14th birthday, and before we even began Kevin announced a surprise: He had added a cake to the day's creations. Already, all of Kevin's equipment seemed to be operating at once. He paused the Robot-Coupe (an industrial food processor) to let us to taste the mango and passionfruit purees that later we'd massage onto Brianna's cake like exotic face creams, so that its pores could absorb the flavor and moisture. He showed us the gemlike edible flowers and berries he had washed with egg whites and dusted in sugar to crystallize. They'd been drying for three days. There was Valrhona chocolate melting in a double boiler on the stovetop, and mixers, ovens, and dehydrators were busy transforming raw materials into delicious components of soon-to-be-breathtaking creations. Brianna was instantly in heaven. She loves to bake. It doesn't matter what it is, if it contains sugar, she has taught herself how to make it. Cakes and cookies are her forte, but she can also make ice cream, elaborate desserts such as Eton mess, and a variety of sweet, indulgent treats. She makes everything entirely from scratch, but she had never tried anything as complex as what she would attempt that day.

As significant as this experience was for her, it was no less so for me. Of all of my food relationships, perhaps none is so complex as that with sugar. I'm willing to bet that it may be the same for you. How many times have you eaten a piece of cake at a birthday party, or a slice of pie during a holiday dinner, and felt like you were "cheating"? How many hours have you spent justifying similar decisions, or beating yourself up over them the next day by limiting your food or adding an extra 20 minutes to your workout? How much mental and emotional energy have you burned just worrying about whether you can get through some special event without "indulging" in the sweets you know will be there?

To some extent, this is because we're faced with undeniable facts about the monster that is sugar in our contemporary food system. Hand in hand with corn — via our old nemesis high-fructose corn syrup — and through other additives such as barley malt, maltose, and malt syrup, sugar is added to a whole host of foods you might not think of as sugary, from ketchup and barbecue sauce to low-fat yogurt and granola. Though sugar fills no nutritional need, we continue to eat it regularly. Even if you adhere to guidelines from the US Department of Agriculture and Department of Health and Human Services and consume no more than 10 percent of your daily calories from sugar, the amount is staggering. For a 2,000-calorie diet, that comes to 200 calories, or about 12 teaspoons. You're thinking, no way I eat 12 teaspoons of sugar every day — that's ¼ cup! And yet, the agencies estimate that the typical American eats about 270 calories of added sugar — about 17 teaspoons' worth — daily. When you consider that one serving of flavored yogurt has 72 calories of added sugars, and one sports drink has about 122 calories of added sugars, you can see how this adds up. And we are daily reminded about the dire health consequences of too much of this stuff: diabetes, heart disease, obesity, to name only a few.

But for me, dealing with sugar has been even more complicated than just coming to grips with its prevalence in our foods. Early in my research into ancestral diets, technologies, and traditional foodways, I became obsessed with how I wanted to feed my young family. From making all of the dairy products we consumed, to hunting and butchering most of our meat, to insisting that no bread but my long-fermented sourdough entered my kids' mouths, I was determined to provide only what I thought were the healthiest foods for our table. To help give my kids foods that resembled what other people were eating—just in a healthier form to make this lifestyle more palatable for them—I made lacto-fermented mayonnaise, ketchup, mustard, and vinegar. I made hot dogs from scratch and even produced cured ham, salami, and mortadella (bologna) so their school lunches didn't look any different from their peers'. For the most part, this was all to the good; my family was eating a nutrient-dense, locally sourced, delicious diet; we were becoming more closely connected to our food; and we were learning and honing important skills.

But there was a dark side. There were entire food categories that I would not eat, and sugar was the biggest and thorniest of all. How many times did I go to a birthday party—even one of our own—and refuse to eat a piece of the cake, no matter how beautifully and thoughtfully prepared? I'd earn the justifiable ire of Christina, so I'd try to placate her by forcing down a single, tiny bite. I became *that guy*. The mental and physical energy that went into tracking down high-quality raw ingredients, making practically everything entirely from scratch, and also serving as the food police so the kids didn't get any "junk" in our house, their grandparents' houses, and even their friends' houses, was all-consuming. I kept convincing myself that no matter how exhausting and stressful it had become, it was worth it. I forced these foods into a special dark place, drawing a rigid and dogmatic divide between what I viewed as good versus bad.

My intentions were heartfelt, but I appeared to be suffering from orthorexia—what the American Psychological Association (APA) defines as "an obsessive concern with eating a healthy or 'pure' diet that is typically very restrictive and more focused on wellness than weight loss. Individuals may insist on eating only certain foods (e.g., those grown locally) or avoid certain food groups... often resulting in extremely low caloric intake, risk of malnutrition, and in extreme cases, death." The APA also notes, "There is some debate about whether orthorexia nervosa is a distinct disorder or a form of anorexia nervosa or obsessive-compulsive disorder." All I know is that I was unknowingly provoking food anxieties and phobias in everyone around me. I may have been meeting my family's biological dietary needs, but I was falling far short in meeting their psychological and emotional needs. Sharing food—the very thing that makes us uniquely human—became filled with anxiety, and nowhere more so than when sweets were in the picture.

When I finally confronted how out of balance my life and my attitude about food had become, I realized something revelatory about everything I had been learning and doing: The healthiest choice isn't always about the food. It's also about who we are as a people, a society, and, in my case, a family. I began to recognize that my unbending approach toward feeding my family didn't allow space for another crucial component of what makes us healthy: the cultural parts of being human. A healthy relationship with food is about much more than merely nutrition. I set out with a new goal that encompassed balancing both components, providing the most nutrient-dense and healthiest food for my family while accepting the cultural demands and expectations of our modern lives. First and foremost, I sought the most nutrient-dense options in any given situation. Then, I looked for homemade options. And I worked to understand the social context of each situation and tried to comprehend the consequences of my actions within each. Finally, I began to ask questions like "Is it worth ingesting sugar to eat this piece of birthday cake my oldest daughter made for my youngest daughter's birthday? Absolutely! Should I feel guilty? Absolutely not!"

Yet, while we make the necessary room for these exceptions, we can and should continue to approach sugar with the same modern hunter-gatherer ethic with which we approach every food in this book, starting with the most basic question: What can I do to make this the safest and most nourishing food it can be? From an ancestral point of view, our modern obsession with—and addiction to—sugar is unhealthy in the extreme. In fact, of all the so-called fringe foods we have talked about in this book, from an ancestral perspective, sugar is the most alien and bizarre of all. Our ancestors had access to only very limited simple carbohydrates. When in rare cases they did acquire sweet things in nature, they were typically in small quantities and only in season, and these natural sweeteners delivered other beneficial nutrients that made eating them worthwhile. The fruits that we find today on our grocery store shelves don't resemble the fruits that our ancestors or even modern hunter-gatherers have access to today. Fruit today is bred to be sweet, often at the expense of other nutrients. This is what the modern food industry is selling us, and what we consumers continue to buy.

Here are just a few examples of the sugar content in fruit: bananas have 18 grams of sugar per cup sliced; cherries 20 grams per cup; pomegranate arils 24 per cup; mangoes 23 per cup sliced; a medium pear has 17 grams; and a medium wedge of watermelon has 17 grams. Compare these to one doughnut at 10 grams; 1 cup of Froot Loops cereal at 12 grams; one 0.6-ounce piece of fudge at 12.4 grams; and 1 cup of Coca-Cola at 27 grams. Dried fruits are even higher because dehydration concentrates the sugar. For example, while 1 cup of grapes contains 15 grams sugar, 1 cup of raisins (dried grapes) contains 106 grams sugar—a 709 percent increase. And finally, remember that while our ancestors ate fruit only when they had access to it, we can eat an imported banana or a bunch of grapes 365 days a year. While certain fruits, such as cherries and pomegranates, usually appear in the grocery store only during certain times of the year, for the most part, seasonality is a myth in the produce section.

In addition to understanding how much sugar is contained in fruit, it is important to understand the sweeteners themselves. Different sweeteners have different tastes, textures, and nutritional profiles, yet our bodies' response to sugar doesn't really discriminate between a tablespoon of table sugar and one of raw honey. They both spike our blood sugar. Table sugar (sucrose) is a disaccharide made up of one glucose molecule and one fructose molecule—so it's 50 percent glucose and 50 percent fructose. The fructose-to-glucose ratios of honey differ depending on variety, but they are similar to that of sucrose.

However, there are other significant differences between sugar and honey that point to which is the healthier sweetener. While sucrose is 100 percent sugar, honey is approximately 85 percent sugar, with the remainder made up of water, minerals, and pollen. Honey's glycemic index ranges from 35 to 74, while sucrose has a glycemic index of 65. Honey also contains vitamins, minerals, and antioxidants, although this can be variable based on how the honey is processed. Most commercial honey today is pasteurized and, as with milk, pasteurization destroys valuable nutrition. Raw honey, on the other hand, is simply filtered, which leaves it alive and full of enzymes and probiotics. Nutrition and chemical composition vary, but raw honey tends to contain vitamins and minerals such as thiamin, niacin, riboflavin, pantothenic acid, calcium, magnesium, manganese, potassium, phosphorus, zinc, vitamin A, vitamin E, and vitamin C. Raw honey's antimicrobial properties help it kill off bad bacteria, yet it also contains prebiotics, food that nourishes the probiotics. Raw honey also contains enzymes that help us digest our food. And, because it includes compounds like flavonoids and phenolic acids, raw honey is a potent antioxidant and anti-inflammatory.

Similarly, there is little in common between pure maple syrup and what is marketed to us as pancake syrup. *Syrup* can mean anything from a mixture of water and sugar to golden syrup or treacle, made from partially refined sugar or molasses. A commercially produced pancake syrup, which is made from corn syrup and a number of chemicals and preservatives, bears no resemblance to pure maple syrup made from the sap of sugar maple trees. While the former has no value as a food, real maple syrup contains inulin—a prebiotic fiber that feeds probiotics—as well as minerals, including calcium, potassium, iron, zinc, and manganese; and antioxidants, including benzoic acid, gallic acid, and cinnamic acid. In 2011, University of Rhode Island researcher Navindra Seeram discovered 34 new beneficial compounds in pure maple syrup and confirmed 20 others that had been discovered the previous year. In the *Journal of Functional Foods,* Seeram and his coauthor, Liya Li, reported that a phenolic compound called quebecol (named after Quebec, the world's leading producer of maple syrup), which researchers did not believe was in sap, is actually produced during the processing of maple syrup. Numerous studies suggest that quebecol effectively kills certain types of cancer cells. And, if the health benefits of maple syrup are not enough, let's not forget the complex, rich, warm taste that can only come from genuine maple syrup.

If we are going to eat something sweet, we might as well use it as an opportunity to take in valuable nutrition—saturated animal fats, protein, minerals, enzymes, vitamins, probiotics, and prebiotics. Combining this dietary strategy with the need for cultural balance, my family has come up with three basic house rules for foods containing sugar: They must be made from scratch, they must be made of the highest-quality ingredients, and they must offer some sort of nutrition so that we are not merely consuming empty calories. (A word here about artificial sweeteners: In my kitchen, they are just not worth it. I would much rather eat a tablespoon of rich maple syrup or raw honey, or even a tablespoon of sugar for that matter, than the equivalent teaspoonful of something created in a lab for the purpose of fooling our senses.) Desserts should have high-quality fat, protein, minerals, vitamins, enzymes, and probiotics and prebiotics whenever possible. These nutrients come from wholesome ingredients—full-fat fermented dairy, eggs from free-roaming chickens that eat plants and insects, and just enough unrefined natural sweeteners (honey, maple syrup, and minimally processed sugars) to provide the sweetness we are looking for.

Which brings us back to the day that Brianna and I spent with Kevin Thornton. Everything we did was focused on sustainability, care, quality, and the joy of connection that is so integral to celebrating and sharing the creation of thoughtful food. We mitigated some of the nutritional issues by cooking with superior ingredients and doing it fully from scratch. Of course, the flour, sugar, eggs, and butter that went into our creations were of the highest quality—we even scraped salt from an enormous block of it that Kevin had collected in Ethiopia and carried home to Ireland—but Kevin took everything up a notch with ingredients he had produced himself. Some, like the passionfruit puree, he had begun to make that same day, while others he had started days or weeks earlier, such as the sugar-and-egg-white-coated dried rose petals and blueberries. One whole wall of his kitchen was a living artwork of shelves displaying jars of ingredients he had been drying, curing, or fermenting for months, and in some cases even years. The vanilla sugar that went into Brianna's cake Kevin made by burying the vanilla pods—the byproduct of removing the seeds to flavor his desserts—in sugar and setting it aside to infuse with all of the vanilla essence. Dried wild plants and leftover vegetable scraps with unique flavor profiles were waiting to be ground precisely when needed (because they are fresher that way), while leftover cake might be ground and included in future dishes to add flavor, color, and texture.

These ingredients also represented Kevin's zero-waste stance in the kitchen. As with the vanilla bean pods buried in sugar, he always tries to find a way to use every bit of his raw materials. Even when our first batch of macarons did not turn out exactly right, rather than tossing them into the compost or rubbish, he set them aside to dehydrate, then crumbled them up and stored them until he could use the "macaron crumble" in something else. We spent the day making sponge cake, gelatins, coulis, garnishes, and macarons. Even Brianna, who had already become our family's resident baker, was fully immersed in the intricate detail, precision, and skill required to create food at this level. And by cooking and learning together, understanding ingredients, and sharing this experience, we fed our emotional needs and our souls. When we left Kevin and climbed back on the train to travel through Dublin back to our cottage, I held on to Brianna as she held on, with two hands, to her exquisite, and exquisitely made, birthday cake.

TIPS AND RECIPES

THE SUGAR BALANCE

Sugar is not good for us. Whether it is glucose, fructose, dextrose, sucrose, or lactose, they all wreak havoc on our bodies. It is important to understand that consuming any simple carbohydrate comes at a cost, but sometimes that cost can be slightly mitigated by choosing foods made with the best ingredients and weighing all factors involved with eating the food. For me, the balance is found in analyzing the following considerations:

1. How much has the sweetener been refined? This directly relates to the type and quantity of nutrients that are present in the sweetener. These can come in the form of minerals, probiotics, prebiotics, vitamins, and even medicinal qualities.
2. What nutrients are delivered through the addition of other ingredients in a dish that help make eating it worthwhile? High-quality egg yolks, milk, and cream can all elevate the nutritional value.
3. What is the social context within which I am eating this? Will eating it help me navigate a social situation, such as a birthday party? What are the cultural and emotional consequences of this decision?
4. Are there other negative consequences to eating this? Will it start an eating binge that will last all day?

TYPES OF SUGAR

All types of sugar are processed at some level, and it is confusing and difficult to tell the difference between them, especially when you are trying to make a healthy decision. The difference, albeit subtle, is whether the sugar was highly processed and how much natural molasses—where the trace minerals such as iron, calcium, magnesium, vitamin B_6, and selenium exist—remains. From a sustainability and ethical perspective, unrefined and raw sugars come from sugar mills that are usually set up at or near sugarcane plantations, while refined sugar is produced at much larger sugar refineries.

Unrefined sugar contains all of the natural molasses and is minimally processed. It can be found at stores or online under names such as muscovado and piloncillo, or the brand Sucanat. If you are going to use sugar, this is the best choice.

Raw sugar is made from juice extracted from the sugarcane, which is then filtered, boiled (no, it is not actually raw), and centrifuged to remove some of the molasses. It retains some natural molasses, but less than unrefined sugar. It can be found under names such as demerara, turbinado, and products like Sugar in the Raw.

Refined sugar comes from sugarcane or sugar beets. It is highly processed in an industrial system that strips the nutrition and uses chemicals such as sulfur dioxide, phosphoric acid, and calcium hydroxide, leaving behind a substance that our bodies are not equipped to handle. Refined sugar includes brown sugar, which is made by artificially replacing some of the molasses that was removed from the refined sugar during processing. While brown sugar is a slightly better choice than plain white sugar, it is similar to drinking milk that has been taken apart and put back together in a food-processing facility. Stay away from refined sugars whenever possible.

CAN CHOCOLATE BE HEALTHY?

Chocolate contains beneficial compounds in the form of flavonoids that are purported to lower cholesterol, reduce inflammation, and prevent blood clots. In fact, some people believe chocolate to be the most powerful antioxidant on the planet. But these benefits come at a cost: All chocolate contains oxalates as well as the toxins caffeine and theobromine; most chocolate is loaded with sugar; and some chocolate contains other ingredients such as emulsifiers and industrial oils. Certainly, some choices are much healthier than others. As with all foods, it all comes down to how the chocolate is processed.

Chocolate comes from seeds of the pods of the cacao tree (*Theobroma cacao*). After they are harvested, the seeds are fermented, dried, roasted, broken into cacao nibs, and winnowed, then ground and melted into cacao liquor. Finally, the cacao liquor is combined with various ingredients that can include sugar, milk powder, cocoa powder, cocoa butter, fats and oils, vanilla, and emulsifiers, to create different products such as milk chocolate, white chocolate, and dark chocolate. Unfortunately, sugar is usually the first ingredient in milk and white chocolate (the latter doesn't even contain cacao liquor or powder; the only ingredient it contains from the cacao tree is cocoa butter). Yet in dark chocolate, sugar is the last ingredient. The number of grams of sugar per 10 grams of white chocolate is 5.7; milk chocolate 5.0; 40 percent dark chocolate 4.0; and 70 percent dark chocolate 2.1. Cacao nibs and cocoa powder are pure cacao and contain no added sugar. Here are the choices (in order) if you want to take advantage of the nutritional benefits of chocolate while keeping added sugars and other ingredients to a minimum:

1. Cacao nibs and pure cocoa powder
2. Dark chocolate (cacao and minimal sugar)
3. Milk chocolate (sugar, milk powder, cacao, and possible other ingredients)

JACQUELINE'S CHOCOLATE MOUSSE

SERVES 4 TO 6

We met the van Wee family in a tiny villa in northern Italy at a weeklong slow food event put together by our dear friends Roeland and Magda Paardekooper in celebration of their 20th wedding anniversary. Véronique van Wee-Barier, the matriarch of the family, generously shared this mousse and their coveted family secret recipe passed down from her mother, Jacqueline Barier. This has since become our family's go-to dessert, and every time we make it we think of the magical week spent making new friends and sharing family recipes made from scratch with fresh, local, seasonal ingredients. I could certainly argue that the protein from the eggs, antioxidants from the chocolate, fat from the butter, and minerals from the unrefined sugar alone make it worth eating. But there is something else less measurable but more important: This recipe, and the memories that making and eating it invoke, are powerful and nourishing in their own right. And isn't that what making and sharing wonderful food is all about?

8 ounces dark chocolate (preferably over 70%)

1 cup Fermented Butter (page 189) or store-bought unsalted butter

8 large eggs

1 cup unrefined sugar (such as Sucanat or muscovado) or raw sugar

1 teaspoon pure vanilla extract

1 cup heavy cream (preferably raw)

Melt the chocolate in a double boiler. Melt the butter in a small saucepan.

Meanwhile, separate the eggs into two large bowls. Beat the egg whites until they form stiff peaks.

Add the sugar and vanilla to the egg yolks and whisk until pale. Add the melted chocolate and melted butter to the yolks and stir to combine. Gently fold the egg whites into the mixture, a spoonful at a time, until thoroughly combined. Refrigerate uncovered for at least 1 hour or, for the best results, overnight.

Just before serving, whip the heavy cream in a bowl until thick. Serve the mousse in bowls topped with a dollop of whipped cream.

HONEY ICE CREAM

Makes about 1½ quarts

This recipe was inspired by a dessert that my friend and master chef Alex Atala serves at his restaurant D.O.M. in São Paulo, Brazil. He finishes the honey ice cream dessert with fermented honey and Amazonian bee pollen. The floral taste of the bee pollen complements the sourness of the honey and the sweet richness of the ice cream perfectly. Bee pollen is available from local beekeepers and online sources, but if you don't have it, don't let that stop you—this is still an amazing dessert without it.

Fermenting the milk and cream harnesses the powerful chemical and physical transformations and predigests the dairy to make it safer and its nutrients more accessible to our bodies. Cooking with egg yolks to create a custard base strikes the perfect balance between flavor, texture, and nutrition, resulting in a dessert my kids love and I feel good about serving them. You can make this recipe by skipping the fermentation step and using either raw or pasteurized milk, but you will be missing out on maximizing the flavor and the nourishing potential of this recipe.

> 2 cups heavy cream (preferably raw)
> 1 cup milk (preferably raw)
> 2 tablespoons Kefir (page 181), Mesophilic Yogurt (page 183),
>   or thermophilic yogurt in a pinch
> 6 large egg yolks
> ¼ teaspoon sea salt
> ½ cup raw honey
> Fermented Honey (page 257), for garnish
> Bee pollen, for garnish (optional)

Pour the cream and milk into a saucepan and slowly warm over low heat, making sure to stir occasionally to avoid burning on the bottom or forming a skin on the top. When it reaches approximately 75°F, it is ready.

Put the kefir or yogurt in a quart-size mason jar. Pour about ½ cup of the warm cream and milk mixture into the jar. Whisk until smooth. This helps make sure the culture is evenly distributed. Pour the rest of the cream and milk mixture into the jar, stir to distribute, cover, and leave in a warm place in your kitchen where it will not be disturbed for 12 to 24 hours.

At the end of the fermentation process, whisk the egg yolks in a medium bowl.

In a heavy saucepan, combine the fermented cream and milk, salt, and raw honey. Slowly bring to a simmer over medium-high heat while stirring to prevent burning.

Once the mixture reaches a simmer, reduce the temperature to medium-low and ladle about ½ cup of the hot mixture into the bowl containing the yolks and whisk to combine. Add another ½ cup of the hot mixture and whisk again.

Pour the warmed yolk mixture back into the hot mixture remaining in the pot. Stir over medium heat until the mixture thickens and coats the back of a spoon.

Prepare an ice-water bath in the sink or in a large bowl. Strain the mixture through a fine-mesh strainer into another medium bowl. Place the bowl in the ice-water bath and let it cool. Cover and refrigerate for several hours or, for the best results, overnight. Churn in an ice cream maker according to the manufacturer's directions.

To serve, scoop into bowls and drizzle a little fermented honey over the top, then finish with a pinch of bee pollen, if you like.

FERMENTED HONEY

The sugars in honey are too concentrated to support fermentation. However, as any beekeeper knows, when the moisture in the honey rises above 19 percent or so, it will spontaneously ferment. In fact, this is how one of the earliest and most famous forms of alcohol is made. Mead, or honey wine (where the word *honeymoon* comes from), is made by diluting raw honey at a ratio of approximately one part honey to five parts water and fermenting it. However, by adding just a little water to bring that moisture content just above 19 percent, we can create a much thicker, mildly fermented honey that is alive with probiotics and has a rich and complex flavor thanks to the lactic acid produced during the fermentation. Use anywhere you would use honey, to top ice cream or even pizza!

1½ cups raw honey
3 tablespoons water

Combine the honey and water in a medium bowl. Stir with a spoon to combine. Pour into a pint-size mason jar and cover loosely with a lid or cheesecloth. Set in a warm place in your kitchen.

Stir daily until the honey shows signs of fermentation — bubbles will appear and a slightly sour and pleasant aroma will arise (this should take about 2 weeks). You don't need to refrigerate this; it will simply stop fermenting, and it can be stored at room temperature for several months.

HEALTHY GUMMIES

Gummies are made with gelatin, which is almost 99 percent protein. Made by cooking collagen, the most plentiful protein in our bodies, gelatin promotes healthy skin, hair, and nails, and it's great for the joints and gut. However, commercial gummies are full of refined sugars and food coloring. If you make them at home, you have complete control over every ingredient, including the type of sweetener used. Avoid using juice from pineapple, kiwi, mango, papaya, or guava, as they contain an enzyme that interferes with the gelatin's ability to set. To make gummy bears (or other shapes), you'll need one or more silicone molds, which are available online.

> 1 cup fresh fruit juice (orange, lemon, lime, etc.)
> 2 tablespoons raw honey or pure maple syrup (optional)
> 2 tablespoons powdered gelatin (preferably from grass-fed cows)
> Avocado or coconut oil, for greasing

Combine the juice and sweetener (if using) in a small saucepan. Stir to combine. Sprinkle the gelatin over the juice and let hydrate (known as "blooming") for about 5 minutes, then whisk until smooth over medium-low heat, until the gelatin has dissolved. (Gelatin that has bloomed will dissolve in liquid at approximately 140°F.) As soon as it has dissolved, immediately remove the pan from the heat and allow to cool slightly before transferring to molds. Overheating gelatin affects its ability to gel, so never let it reach a boil.

While the fruit juice is cooling, lightly grease a small baking pan or silicone mold with avocado or coconut oil. If using a silicone mold, transfer the cooled but still warm mixture to a squeeze bottle, then fill the mold; otherwise just pour the gelatin mixture into the baking pan. Refrigerate for at least 6 hours or overnight, until the mixture fully sets. Once it has set, pop the gummies out of the mold, or cut them in the pan into cubes. The gummies can be stored in an airtight container in the fridge for several weeks.

CHOCOLATE MAPLE SOURDOUGH CAKE WITH GANACHE

MAKES 1 CAKE

Cake plays a central role in this chapter and is often the key element in so many social functions. There are many reasons to eat cake, but biological health is not one of them. There is no such thing as a "healthy" cake, and no one eats cake to get healthier. However, there are ways to make cake as healthy as possible and still create a product that is beautiful, delicious, and a pleasure to eat. In this recipe, I have used a sourdough approach to transform the wheat into its safest and most nourishing form possible, relied on maple syrup to sweeten the cake, made use of a Bundt cake shape so that there is no need for an unhealthy filling, and topped it all with dark chocolate ganache to avoid the excess sugar that would be found in other frostings.

225 grams (1 cup) mature sourdough mother culture
  (see page 128)
240 grams (1 cup plus 1 tablespoon) milk
240 grams (2 cups) all-purpose flour, plus more for dusting
227 grams (1 cup) Fermented Butter (page 189) or store-bought
  unsalted butter, room temperature, plus more for greasing
316 grams (1 cup) pure maple syrup
9 grams (2 teaspoons) pure vanilla extract
100 grams (1 cup) unsweetened cocoa powder
9 grams (1½ teaspoons) baking soda
5 grams (1 teaspoon) sea salt
2 large eggs
228 grams (8 ounces) dark chocolate (preferably over 70%),
  chopped or in chips
230 grams (1 cup) heavy cream

Combine the sourdough mother, milk, and flour in a medium bowl. Stir to thoroughly combine (a Danish dough whisk is the perfect tool for this). Cover and allow to ferment at room temperature (about 75°F) overnight (or approximately 12 hours).

The next day, preheat the oven to 350°F. Grease a 10- or 12-cup Bundt pan with butter and dust with flour.

To the sourdough mixture, add the softened butter, maple syrup, vanilla, cocoa powder, baking soda, and salt and mix with a stand mixer or hand mixer until all ingredients are incorporated. Add the eggs, one at a time, and continue mixing until smooth.

Pour the batter into the prepared pan and bake for 45 minutes, or until a toothpick inserted in the center of the cake comes out clean. Allow to cool in the pan slightly for 15 minutes, then invert onto a cooling rack. Cool thoroughly before adding the ganache.

Put the dark chocolate in a medium heatproof bowl. Pour the cream into a small saucepan and bring to a simmer over low heat. When it reaches a simmer, pour the hot cream over the dark chocolate and cover the bowl with a plate for 5 minutes. After 5 minutes, remove the plate and stir to melt any remaining chocolate pieces until smooth. Allow to cool a little longer to achieve a thicker consistency that is just barely pourable, about 15 minutes.

Slowly pour the ganache over the cake so that it is evenly distributed. Allow the ganache to fully cool before serving. Cover leftovers and store at room temperature for up to 3 days.

CONCLUSION

If there is one single lesson to learn from our hunter-gatherer ancestors, it is how to make the most of any situation — in other words, how to adapt. And while it's important for us to understand our ancestral dietary past as it relates to our biological and physical needs — then and now — we can't do it in a vacuum. We can't exclude all of the other reasons we need to eat and drink, and how so many of those reasons are intricately entwined with everything it means to be human: identity, family, tradition, religion, sense of place, nationalism, environmental ethics. To be truly healthy, we have to embrace all sides of this very human equation. We need to continue to maximize our foods' nutrient density and bioavailability to make us biologically healthy, while fully supporting our cultural health by making food that is pleasing to our modern palates and sense of aesthetics, then sharing, gathering, and enjoying this food with one another.

Both of these considerations must be weighed as we move through this food landscape as modern hunter-gatherers. Extremism doesn't work, as I learned all too well. We would never be able to maintain our busy, modern, full-time working lives and hunt, gather, fish, trap, ferment, grind, cook, cure, and bake all of our food, even if the resources were there and we had the skill sets to do so. Instead, we need to be honest with ourselves. We need to realize what is truly important to us, to compromise in the space that realization provides, and to build meaningful lives and diets within those contexts. There is no one-size-fits-all approach. It is individual and contextual, and it requires work and commitment.

And this is where I encourage you not to be overwhelmed. We are all coming at this from different places geographically, emotionally, economically, philosophically. Some of you may want to adopt some form of everything we've talked about in this book. Others may be happy with making pancakes from scratch on a Sunday morning rather than reaching for a box of mix. Small, consistent, lasting changes are difficult to quantify, but they are more powerful than you can imagine. Even the slightest of changes, compounded over a long period of time, can have enormous impact. Think about this: What if you made just one loaf of genuine sourdough bread each week, and every sandwich your child took to school was made from that bread? That's approximately 2,340 sandwiches (or almost 5,000 slices of bread) over the average American kid's K–12 school career. That's 2,340 opportunities for your child to eat a food that maximizes nutrition and bioavailability—and that came from your own hands and heart—rather than a store-bought, processed, nutritionally bereft, artificially fortified and flavored alternative. That weekly loaf of bread translates into meaningful, long-term change in your child's health, and in how you reclaim your agency in this complicated, confusing modern foodscape.

Becoming a more educated consumer is crucial, so when you walk into a grocery store, you see with fresh, informed eyes and make the healthiest choices you can. Pioneering food traditions are built during times of need, and we find ourselves in one of the greatest dietary predicaments of our history as humans. We must forge innovative traditions that balance our ancestral biological requirements with our modern cultural needs to create genuine health in ourselves, our families, our communities, and our world. And this food revolution begins in your own kitchen, and around your table.

ACKNOWLEDGMENTS

My life has taken an unconventional path, one that for many years seemed to have no clear direction. My relationship with food began badly and got worse through high school and college. My education was sidelined when I went blind as a result of an eye disease, keratoconus. Throughout, I snuck in as much foraging, hunting, primitive technologies, cooking, and archaeology as I could, never knowing how they could be anything more than disparate interests. Only later did I learn that they could work synergistically to become the lens through which I view the world, and that they would form the foundation for my work and, by extension, this book.

I never could have navigated this difficult road without the many people who have helped me along the way. I am honored to have the opportunity to thank you publicly, here.

To the families who made the decision to declare their loved ones — in the final moments of their lives — organ donors and enabled me to receive two corneal transplants. I cannot imagine how difficult it must have been to be so generous during such a heartbreaking time. I have literally seen the world through your loved ones' eyes. And to Dr. Theodore Perl, the talented surgeon who performed the corneal transplant surgery. All of you gave me the gift of sight and changed my life. Thank you.

To Coach David Icenhower, who moved mountains to get me accepted into the College of New Jersey (TCNJ) — despite my having both failed out and dropped out of the Ohio State University (yes, you read that right) — by using my remaining eligibility to wrestle for his program. At TCNJ, I met my wife, Christina, and ultimately graduated after declaring eight different majors throughout my 10-year undergraduate career. I also received my first meaningful academic advising when members of the

History Department took a genuine interest in me and my future and even helped support and guide my decision to go to graduate school.

To Dr. R. Michael Stewart and the entire Temple University Anthropology Department, who took a chance and accepted me into their graduate program when others told me that I was not graduate-school material, and that I should just be content to have graduated college and landed a job.

To my students around the world—whether from an academic institution like Hillsborough High School, Temple University, Monmouth University, University College Dublin (UCD), and Washington College, or through a virtual cooking class or foraging tour—thank you for challenging me and giving me a reason always to push, to conduct new research, and to find ways to translate what I learn into something I can share in the classroom, no matter what form that classroom takes.

To the people who have helped me define the foundation of my education and teaching, an approach that incorporates archaeology (to learn about the past), primitive technology (hands-on work with ancient skills), and experimental archaeology (applying primitive technology skills using the scientific method to interpret the archaeological record). I have been fortunate to have trained under mentors including Jack Cresson, Dr. Errett Callahan, and Dr. Maria Sidoroff, and to work with colleagues including Dr. Roeland and Magda Paardekooper, Dr. Tim Messner, Laurent Mazet, Dr. Javier Baena, Kirk Drier, Are Tsirk, Scott Silsby, Steve Nissly, Peter Viking, Dr. Linda Hurcombe, Dr. Seamus Caufield, Dr. Aidan O'Sullivan, Dr. Brendan O'Neil, Dr. John Seidel, Liz Seidel, Dr. Rich Veit, Steve Adams, Barry Adrian and Dr. Nick Dixon, Pascale Barnes, Diederik Pomstra, Mark Butler, Steve Watts, Doug Meyer, Dr. Berit Eriksen, Steven Fox, Mike Frank, Greg High, Scott Jones, Dr. Greg Lattanzi, Dr. Theresa Kamper, and Dr. Marianne Rasmussen. Thank you also to the organizations that have given me a home, inspired me, and created an opportunity to network with other researchers: EXARC, REARC, MAAC, and the open-air museum Lejre: Land of Legends.

To the remarkable chefs and revolutionaries in the food world, who have been such incredible sources of information and inspiration: Chef John Nocita, Juan Penzini, Mariana Brewer, Dawn DeStefano, and the entire

Italian Culinary Institute family around the world, Chef Alex Atala, Chef Kevin Thornton and Muriel Thornton, Sandor Katz, David Asher, Wayne Caddy, Michael Pollan, Stef De Haan, Rigel Sotelo, Cliffe Arrand, Sally Fallon Morrell, Lierre Keith, Kirk Lombard, Sally Norton, Brian Sanders, Dr. Gary Shlifer, and Hilda Gore.

To National Geographic and the *Great Human Race* crew for keeping me safe and helping create an experience of a lifetime that shaped so much of my work and the manner in which I view the past. A huge thank-you to Brandon Gulish, Pete DeLasho, Brian Lovett, Cat Bigney, Kevin Hoban, Anneli Gericke, Griffin Kenemer, Tahria Sheather, Luke Cormack, Burt Gregory, Brent Meske, Jovan Sales, Jesse Brooks, and Todd Curtis.

To the people around the world who have opened their homes and shared their hearths, tables, and vast knowledge with me and my family: Galia Kleiman and Enrique Tron, Rigel Sotelo, Delia and Andy Stirling, Sophie and Calum Macfarlane, Sue and Dave Brown, Emiliano Ramirez Lopez and Maria Francisca Bautista Martines (Juana), Giacinto Cangelosi, Francisco Huanca Samo, Juana Colque Jallasi, Carmen Huanca Colque, Catalina Huanca Colque, Helmut Poschel, Konrad Knopp, Milka Tello, Marc Brown, Markus Shimizu, Massimo Reverberi, David Pattison, the Kongelai Village in West Pokot, Boonchoo Kitsantria, his family, and his village. Thank you. I am honored to share your stories.

To the people who supported my research and work and helped provide it a voice to reach a larger audience. Among them are Larry and Wendy Culp, Ann Horner, John McCray, Richard and Jane Creighton, Rick and Kathleen Wheeler, Brandon Riker, University College Dublin, Shay Kendrick of Compass Group, Odaios Foods, Dr. Emily Chamlee-Wright, Wayne Hendricks, Ted Maris-Wolf, Steve and Somers Fullerton, Doug Rae, Daryl L. Swanstrom, Washington College faculty and staff, Bonny Wolf, Peppo Marotta, Evelin Faustino Damian, Siddharta Altamirano, Deborah Moye, Joe Spinelli, Tamara Kerr, Kathy Smith-Wenning, Nathan Preteseille, Noah Kegley, and Dr. Briana Pobiner. Thank you.

To the people who made this book a reality. I remember vividly the day I decided to write a book. It was the moment my seventh-grade English teacher returned a writing assignment and told me that despite my love for writing, I should give it up and find something else to do. Making this book happen was nothing short of a miracle. Seven years have passed since I typed the first words of the original manuscript and the day I submitted the final version for publication. Throughout this process, I have learned the value in being surrounded by a talented team of people and have witnessed, firsthand, what they can create when focused around delivering a powerful message. Deborah Grosvenor, my literary agent, for seeing a spark of hope in this book and finding it such a perfect home. Tracy Behar and her team at Little, Brown, for realizing the value in this project, and for her support and guidance and being such an absolute pleasure to work with. Wendy Mitman Clarke, for being nothing short of a miracle worker. A talented writer, editor, colleague, and friend, she single-handedly transformed my academic prose and tangled threads of crazy ideas into a message that is clear, relevant, and accessible. Thank you for your patience, your perseverance, and for working your magic. Outside readers Shane Brill and Roberta Hilbruner, who read and reread draft after draft to ensure the information was as accurate and accessible as possible. Illustrator Sarah Schlick, whose sketches made difficult steps in the text easier to understand. My photographer, Brianna Schindler, who made these dishes come alive through her gorgeous photographs. And lawyers Stewart Barroll, Steve McAuliffe, and Mitra Ahouraian, who made the legalese work to make this happen. Thank you all for believing in me, my family, and this project.

Finally, to family, both immediate and far-flung. To everyone in Ireland, where most of the research for this book took place, thank you for embracing our family and sharing your beautiful country. Our experience was so intense and the bonds we created so strong that we consider you all family — our St. Olaf's family, Bronzeman/Belderrig family, University College Dublin family, and Airfield family. And a huge thank-you to our dear friend and adventure companion Jason O'Brien, who has a gift for making global connections and bringing people together over the most meaningful of meals. To Jim Burden, Paul Eberhardt, and James Carlos Smith (Smitty), the adventures we shared decades ago planted the seeds for so much of what I do now. Thank you for a lifetime of friendship.

ACKNOWLEDGMENTS

I fully realize that I would have not been able to accomplish anything meaningful in my life without my immediate family. No matter how many times I have stumbled, they have been a constant source of love, support, and guidance. My mother and father, Bill and Barrie Schindler, instilled in me a passion for the outdoors, a love for the kitchen, and a keen interest in the past. My father taught me to hunt, trap, and fish, and my mother taught me to cook and understand the importance of food as nourishment. Together they showed me how to work with my hands, the merit of hard work, and what is most valuable in life; they modeled love and the importance of family. I didn't know it then, but all of this laid the foundation for how and why I conduct my research. Thank you.

My mother- and father-in-law, Jane and Steve Nightingale, have also been a constant source of support since they met me, from pulling over and letting me jump out of the car no matter where we were headed because I saw a plant on the side of the road in desperate need of identification, or taking in me and Christina to live with them as poor graduate students so that we could save money and concentrate on school. Thank you.

To my sister, Heather Freeman, brother-in-law, Michael Nightingale, and their families — every family camping trip, hike, and even marathon game of Monopoly have helped shaped my world. Thank you.

To my kids, Brianna, Billy, and Alyssa. Thank you for making our family complete. You are the inspiration for everything I do, and I am so incredibly proud of each of you. Thank you for being my taste testers, traveling companions, and sources of inspiration. Our family's journey to learn to Eat Like Humans is the journey that has culminated in this book.

To my wife, Christina, thank you for being my everything. The research required to write this book would not have been possible without you sharing my belief in the importance of feeding our family the most nourishing food possible, and your crazy, wild, adventurous spirit that allowed our family to explore and thrive in any situation anywhere in the world. This book is the result of your love, support, hard work, and tech skills. I couldn't imagine a more amazing partner, wife, and friend. I love you completely.

RECIPE INDEX

RECIPE INDEX

INDEX

ABOUT THE AUTHOR

Dr. Bill Schindler is an internationally known archaeologist, primitive technologist, and chef. He founded and directs the Eastern Shore Food Lab with a mission to preserve and revive ancestral dietary approaches to create a nourishing, ethical, and sustainable food system and is an adjunct associate professor of archaeology at University College Dublin. His work is currently the focus of *Wired* magazine's YouTube series, *Basic Instincts* and *Food Science,* and he co-starred in the National Geographic Channel series *The Great Human Race,* which aired in 2016 in 171 countries. Dr. Schindler has also been featured on CNN, Maryland Public Television, NPR's *Weekend Edition* and *Here and Now,* as well as on such podcasts as *Milk Street Radio, Peak Human,* and *The Academic Minute.* Dr. Schindler's work has appeared in the *Washington Post, The Atlantic,* and the London *Times,* among other publications.